WHEN WE COLLIDE

SEX,
SOCIAL RISK,
AND
JEWISH
ETHICS

REBECCA J. EPSTEIN-LEVI

INDIANA UNIVERSITY PRESS

This book is a publication of

Indiana University Press
Office of Scholarly Publishing
Herman B Wells Library 350
1320 East 10th Street
Bloomington, Indiana 47405 USA

iupress.org

© 2023 by Rebecca J. Epstein-Levi

Manufactured in the United States of America

First printing 2023

Library of Congress Cataloging-in-Publication Data

Names: Epstein-Levi, Rebecca J., author.
Title: When we collide : sex, social risk, and Jewish ethics / Rebecca J.
  Epstein-Levi.
Description: Bloomington, Indiana : Indiana University Press, 2023. |
  Series: New Jewish philosophy and thought | Includes bibliographical
  references and index.
Identifiers: LCCN 2022024556 (print) | LCCN 2022024557 (ebook) | ISBN
  9780253064998 (hardback) | ISBN 9780253065001 (paperback) | ISBN
  9780253065018 (ebook)
Subjects: LCSH: Sex—Religious aspects—Judaism. | Sexual ethics. | Jewish
  ethics. | Rabbinical literature—History and criticism.
Classification: LCC BM720.S4 E617 2023 (print) | LCC BM720.S4 (ebook) |
  DDC 296.3/6—dc23/eng/20220608
LC record available at https://lccn.loc.gov/2022024556
LC ebook record available at https://lccn.loc.gov/2022024557

FOR SARAH,
who keeps me vulnerable and thereby keeps me kind

FOR KATHRYN,
who by her example as a Christian taught me how to be a Jew.

AND FOR MY WHOLE CHOSEN FAMILY,
*who are at once a wonderful, mad, unruly community
and yet one of a kind, no category.*

CONTENTS

ACKNOWLEDGMENTS

THIS BOOK DEVELOPED OUT of my dissertation (University of Virginia, 2017), "Safe, Sane, and Attentive: Toward a Jewish Ethic of Sex and Public Health," and chapters 1 and 4 in particular draw heavily on the work I did in it. It also means that I owe debts of gratitude to the many people who helped me complete that project, beginning with my director, Margaret Mohrmann. Margaret's encouragement, mentorship, formidable editorial powers, and, above all, friendship have helped me develop into a far better and more rigorous scholar than I otherwise would be, and her sense of humor has helped me remember not to take myself too seriously. The other members of my committee—Elizabeth Shanks Alexander, Beth Epstein, and Peter Ochs—also played critical roles in the development of this project and in my development as a scholar. Peter Ochs, perhaps more than anyone else, has shaped me as a Jewish reasoner, and it is thanks to his intense and prophetic love for the never-ending dance between living text, engaged interpretation, and inspired practice that I have learned to work with texts as genuine partners. Elizabeth Shanks Alexander—also a formidable editrix—has taught me invaluable hermeneutic rigor. Thanks to Liz, I know the importance of a clear and focused pair of reading glasses for the construction and proper use of strong and effective riot gear. And I am deeply grateful for Beth Epstein's kindness, encouragement, and relentlessly practical focus. Others in the Religion Department at UVA who contributed immeasurably to this project and to my development as a scholar include Asher Biemann, Larry Bouchard, Jim Childress, Martien Halvorson-Taylor, Willis Jenkins, Charles Mathewes, Karl

Shuve, and Liz Smith. Special mention must go to Professor Vanessa Ochs, who is my rabbi and friend as well as my professor, and to Nichole Flores, whose insights in conversation have enriched the project and who has also become a dear friend. So too must thanks be given to my friends and cohorts: Deborah Barer, Mark Randall James, and Kathryn Ray read and commented on substantial sections of this work at various stages of drafting, and my work is richer and more rigorous for their insights. Conversations with Ashleigh Elser, Nauman Faizi, Kelly Figueroa-Ray, Emily Filler, Charlie Gillespie, Paul Gleason, Joe Lenow, and Daniel Wise also developed and refined my arguments in important ways.

Thanks are also due to colleagues at Oberlin College, where I taught while I finished the dissertation: Cindy Chapman, Martino Dibeltulo Concu, Cheryl Cottine, Rabbi Megan Doherty, Laura Herron, David Kamitsuka, Margaret Kamitsuka, Tamika Nunley, Abe Socher, Sarah Pierce Taylor, and Danielle Terrazas Williams. Particular thanks go to Chip Lockwood, without whose encouragement and accountability during our Wednesday morning writing dates I would have been far harder pressed to finish on time.

As the project began its long metamorphosis from dissertation to book, I continued to draw on the invaluable guidance of Margaret Mohrmann and Liz Alexander, who read significant parts of the book manuscript at various points and provided both critical insight, invaluable support, and incredibly warm and lovely cheerleading as I developed the project from a dissertation to a full-fledged book. Dear friends both inside the academy and out also read and discussed parts of this book at various stages in its development and provided invaluable feedback. Particular thanks are due to Laura Alexander, Wendy Love Anderson, Deborah Barer, Jessica Belasco, Julia Watts Belser, Fannie Bialek, Becca Colmer, Emily Filler, Bramble Graham, Alyssa Henning, Carly Palans, Michal Raucher, Kathryn Ray, Ruti Regan, and Vesper. Y'all are one of a kind, no category.

Thanks are also due to the students in various iterations of my Jewish Sexual Ethics course at Oberlin College, Washington University in St. Louis, and Vanderbilt University, who read and discussed parts of the manuscript at various stages in its development. This book is richer and more thoughtful for their input. And my mentors and cohorts in the Sacred Writes Public Scholarship Training Fellowship—Vicki Brennan, Elizabeth Bucar, Brian Clites, Alison Melnick Dyer, Shreena Gandhi, Megan Goodwin, Sajida Jalalzai,

Brett Krutzch, Tia Noelle Pratt, and Kayla Reneé Wheeler—helped me fully understand and articulate the public appeal and import of my project.

I drafted the vast majority of the manuscript during my tenure as the Friedman Postdoctoral Fellow in Jewish Studies at Washington University in St. Louis (2017–2019), which gave me the time, resources, and space necessary to do this work. I'm grateful to my mentors and colleagues there, especially Wendy Love Anderson, Pamela Barmash, Nancy Berg, Fannie Bialek, Martin Jacobs, Hillel Kieval, Aria Nakisa, Nancy Reynolds, Stephen Scordias, Lesile Smith, and Vasiliki Touhouliotis. As I've finalized the manuscript from my current position at Vanderbilt University, I'm also infinitely grateful for the support I've received from my colleagues here, especially my amazing chairs, Katherine Crawford and Allison Schachter, who have been incredible advocates for me. Thanks are also due to Julia Cohen, Elizabeth Reeves Covington, Sydney Grimes, Barbara Kaeser, Shaul Kelner, Stacy Clifford Simplican, and Danyelle Valentine.

The project would have been, of course, impossible without Gary Dunham, Anna Francis, Ashante Thomas, and Darja Malcolm-Clarke at Indiana University Press (IUP), as well as Megan Schindele at Amnet and indexer Melissa Stearns Hyde. I'm massively grateful to Zachary Braiterman, in his role as series editor for the New Jewish Philosophy and Thought series at IUP for expressing interest in the manuscript and shepherding it through the processes of submission and review, and to the invaluable guidance I received from my anonymous reviewers. Additionally, Martin Kavka provided invaluable, gimlet-eyed—and *hilarious*—support and editorial insight throughout this stage, and I genuinely don't know where I'd be on the project without him. And a *massive* cheer for Meli Sameh, who did brilliant work formatting the final manuscript, assembling the bibliography, and standardizing my, ah, creative transliterations.

I couldn't have written this book without the best of feline companionship— ably and adorably provided by Faintly Macabre and Chroma the Great. By stealing my pens and bookmarks, threatening to shred wayward notepapers, and attacking typing fingers, Faintly forces me to be alert, self-aware, and conscious of my surroundings in a way that I hope would elicit at least faint recognition and approval from the rabbis of the Mishnah. And her boldness and willingness to frankly assert her needs is a fine model indeed for those of us who have been socialized to be habitually deferential (although her consideration of the needs of others could still use a bit of work). Chroma, meanwhile—with her unfailingly sweet nature; adorable squeaks, chirps, and burbles; and impossibly soft fur—is an utter ray of light who can be counted on to relieve stress and put things in perspective when nothing else can. Really, all writers (who like cats and aren't insurmountably allergic to them) who can have cats should.

And, of course, no acknowledgment would be complete without Sarah Epstein-Levi, whose love, support, and practical assistance have played a key role in making this book what it is. Sarah's psychological knowledge and scientific sensibilities have helped me navigate the research necessary to ground this project in solid empirical data. Sarah taught me how to read a scientific paper and pointed me toward several of the bodies of research I would go on to use here; at critical times she also turned her powers of research toward helping me fill holes in my references. Even more importantly, her care, intelligence, and humor have kept me sane and grounded throughout the process. I love you, Starling.

WHEN WE COLLIDE

INTRODUCTION

SEX DOES NOT OCCUR in a moral vacuum. It exists in physical, psycho-logical, and moral contiguity to other social interactions. Its attendant plea-sures, risks, and rituals shape individuals and the multiple communities they constitute in ways that are inextricably entangled with the structures, norms, choices, and accidents that create the conditions for flourishing or its oppo-site, the conditions that make lives livable or not. To give a proper moral ac-count of sex and to generate liberatory sexual norms, therefore, one must pay close attention to its messy details and to the ways those details are shared with other collisions of the flesh and psyche. Rabbinic texts—with their atten-tion to the granular details of social risk and contagion, their troubled medita-tions on power dynamics at both interpersonal and international levels, and their careful and sometimes unexpected understanding of the relationships between individual self-examination and self-formation and the structures of communal norms—can be unique and valuable resources for this project. But they can only do so justly in dialogue with voices that give clear, detailed, and generous empirical accounts of the lives, rituals, and moral priorities of real sexual actors.

There is no shortage of material, whether it be scholarly, homiletic, liter-ary, confessional, or something else, on religious sexual ethics. Even within the realms of Jewish thought, my bookshelves and hard drive are filled with materials that offer a range of perspectives on the whys, whethers, and where-fores of how the children of Israel ought to engage with one another's naughty bits. And narrowing the field even further, there is a considerable body of

1

Jewishly connected literature that gets at some aspect of these questions from feminist and queer standpoints. So why does the field require yet another treatise from an angry, neurodivergent queer woman (or whatever other constellation of identities) arguing for some kind of apparently liberalized or queered approach to sexual ethics?

The answer to this question is that systems of religious ethics have struggled to deal with sex in ways that adequately account for its empirical realities. Our normative claims about sexuality reveal truths about our descriptive claims regarding sexuality—truths that, furthermore, may belie our *rhetoric* regarding our descriptive claims. On the face of it, for example, my claim that sex is intertwined with other forms of social interaction is hardly a novel one even within the field of religious ethics: indeed, even the most restrictive of sexual ethicists couch their prescriptions in the language of upholding broader social and communal order. It is my claim, however, that many of these writers are paying lip service to the *idea* of sex as a social phenomenon while in fact treating it quite differently than they treat any other form of social interaction. That is to say, their rhetoric of sexuality is not congruent with their treatment of it in practice, which restricts sexual expression to specific classes of people and extols abstinence for everyone else on the grounds of sex's attendant risks in ways that are not consistent with their treatment of other social risk activities.

In this, Judaism is no exception. While *halakhic* discourse has addressed practical questions of sex and sexuality throughout its existence, Jewish sexual ethics as a modern discipline is a fairly recent phenomenon—not only because the same is true regarding the academic discipline of Jewish ethics generally but also because modern and contemporary sexual ethics grapples with questions that would have been unthinkable to the framers of halakhic discourse. Thus, while Conservative and Orthodox *poskim* (halakhic decisors) continue to field questions about practical sexual matters, the academic analysis of those practical matters is, at best, limited. Further, there exists a frustrating divide in what little academic writing exists on the subject: voices that are willing to address specific, practical questions tend to be conservative and relatively uninformed by feminist and queer thought; conversely, voices that are attentive to feminist and queer thought tend to be far less interested in precisely those specific, practical questions, preferring to focus on broader, more theoretical questions of gender and sexuality writ large—that is to say, they are about gender and sexuality more broadly construed and only incidentally about sexual ethics as such.[1]

There are two major underlying components of this problem. First, within academic Jewish sexual ethics, at least, sex *as an empirical, lived, and granular phenomenon* is a seriously underanalyzed category. Jewish scholars have spent much time on sex as a theoretical phenomenon, asking what it tells us about God, creation, prayer, human nature, and so on. They have spent even more time thinking about sex as a distinguishing phenomenon, one that sets Judaism apart from other traditions in significant ways—it is noteworthy, for example, that regardless of how restrictive or permissive, cautious or expansive, a modern Jewish ethicist is about sexuality, they will almost always aver that Judaism as a tradition is notably sexually affirming, certainly far more so than Christianity.[2] However, with the exception of Jennie Rosenfeld's excellent but unpublished dissertation, there is not, to my knowledge, a systematic, book-length Jewish treatment of sex that offers a sustained moral analysis of particular lived sexual experiences.

Second, it is nearly ubiquitous within the field of Jewish ethics for the primary source of particular moral norms to come out of classical rabbinic sources. Even bracketing the problematics of relying on these sources to the exclusion of Jews' lived experiences, the prevailing hermeneutic in this field has recently come under significant and, to my mind, justified criticism.[3] Too often, Jewish ethicists employ a method by which they look for simplistic one-to-one topical correspondence between the contemporary problem they are evaluating and the subject matter of a given rabbinic text. This kind of "proof texting" elides social, literary, and historical complexities of the text and its world, and it tends to produce a parallel oversimplification of the contemporary problem at hand. Perhaps unsurprisingly, this tendency to proof text has been a particularly common problem within the subfield of Jewish sexual ethics. Writers tend to refer to a small set of classical texts whose subject matter appears *explicitly* sexual, and this becomes the increasingly overdrawn well from which flows contemporary Jewish sexual ethics.

This book addresses both of these components by beginning with the premise that sex, rather than being a sui generis phenomenon, is a species of social interaction that is contiguous and entangled with other species of social interactions. It is thus not possible to separate any treatment of sex—moral treatments very much included—from the ways we treat other forms of social interaction. And, as I shall argue below, this inability to separate sex from its larger social context has a number of implications, chief among which are that it forces consideration of the particulars of sex as a lived experience and that it expands and enriches the range of textual resources available to the Jewish ethicist.

Core Claims, Foundational Concepts, and Dialogue Partners

This book is a project in Jewish virtue ethics, by which I mean that I use Jewish texts as dialogue partners for thinking about how sex shapes individuals and communities as moral actors. Its fulcral claim is that sex is not sui generis but is rather a species of social intercourse that is contiguous and intertwined with other species of social intercourse. Sexual relations are not even as *descriptively* separable from other forms of social relations as we might think—business transactions, casual conversations, professional relationships, and friendships can all be sexually charged, while primarily sexual interactions are almost always colored by nonsexual social relationships, interactions, and norms. This claim is hardly news to the fields of women's, gender, and sexuality studies and queer studies, but it is one that is badly underaccounted for in the field of religious ethics. And this is a problem, because the claim that sex is a species of social intercourse that is intertwined with other species of the same has radically significant moral implications. The ways we behave sexually reflect and affect the ways we behave in other social situations; the sorts of risks and benefits we encounter in sexual relations are the same sorts of risks and benefits we encounter in other kinds of social relations—the ways we are shaped as individuals, the ways we form and are formed by communities, and the moral claims our fellows and our communities make upon us and vice versa.

Compass Points: Key Concepts

Some key concepts help draw out the contours and implications of this claim. First, there is *empirical pertinence*, which means, simply enough, that anything or anyone—a text, a practice, a decision, a person, a community—that one might seek to interpret has real, tangible qualities that matter both for their own sakes and to the ways one interprets them. Interpreters have a duty to attend to these empirical realities in detail, to consider them within their contexts, and to make a good-faith effort to hear and take seriously their interlocutors' self-accounting. *Risk,* which is inherent in all interactions, including interpretive ones, is the relative probability that some unpleasant or harmful outcome may occur, either along with or instead of some neutral or beneficial outcome. *Community,* which at one level is a method of managing risk, refers to both (1) a general obligation to the collective well-being and the recognition that our welfare is bound up in that of our fellows' and (2) specific collectives formed around shared affinities that form the members and the collective in distinct and characteristic ways. *Formation*—also at one level a method of managing risk—refers to the ways our practices, beliefs, and social and material contexts mold us into specific ways of being and not others, through both direct and explicit and indirect and implicit means. *Diversity* here refers to a potentially infinite range of practices and ways of being that are morally valuable in themselves but that communities can struggle to accommodate and often actively suppress, in large part because heterogeneity increases some kinds of risk. Finally, the goal of all these things, *livability,* is a state of dynamic balance among one's own needs and desires, the needs and desires of individual others with whom one interacts, and the basic structures of the social orders in which one lives such that flourishing is accessible to everyone and that no one experiences unbearable hardship.

To elucidate these key concepts and apply them to my project of a normative sexual ethic, I engage several key dialogue partners. Classical rabbinic texts offer fresh and unexpected ways of approaching all these concepts. But as much recent scholarship in rabbinics has demonstrated, if these texts are not themselves approached with a great deal of interpretive care and attention to empirical pertinence, they risk reinscribing stale and oppressive norms and patterns of thought. Crip and critical disability studies offer crucial reexaminations of the value of diverse ways of being, of questions of appropriate risk management and of just who is allowed to manage and undertake risks, and of the fluid parameters of livability. And anthropologies of particular sexual communities offer empirical resources necessary for engaging sex and sexual diversity as the lived social interactions they are with appropriate interpretive care.

Dialogue Partners: Rabbinic Texts

Since I work within a Jewish religious, moral, and textual tradition, my first and most obvious dialogue partners in this project are classical rabbinic texts. These texts have been, as I noted above, the major source of moral norms both for systems of halakhah and for the much younger discipline of academic Jewish ethics. Broadly speaking, engaging with these texts thus links my own project with long-standing traditions of Jewish moral and textual reasoning. The specific texts I engage with at length in this book offer particular resources for a liberatory sexual ethic. The story of the tempestuous relationship between Rabbi Yoḥanan and Resh Laḳish in Bavli Bava Metsia 84a offers an ultimately tragic portrait both of the serious risks inherent in social, emotional, and intellectual intimacy and of the life-giving character of those very risks. Selections from Mishnah Zavim invite us to rethink our collective attitudes toward and management strategies for socially transmitted contagion. The "Oven of Akhnai" narrative in Bava Metsia 59a–b, as well as several selections from Mishnah Sanhedrin, put in dialogue with present-day BDSM communities, offer a model for a community formed around a risk activity that is intended to shape members in specific ways, while also navigating the implications of occupying liminal positions of power. And the tragic story of Ḥaruta and Rabbi Ḥiyya bar Ashi in Bavli Ḳidushin 81b shows us some of the ways sex is inseparable from broader social ethics and intimately ties the importance of attending to empirical pertinence and to the duties we owe one another as social actors.

These texts do not, however, always offer these resources in straightforward or obvious ways. Interpretive care is crucial to this enterprise, and along these lines, I make a significant hermeneutic claim throughout this book, which I discuss in detail in chapter 1. As I discuss above, the prevailing hermeneutic within academic Jewish ethics, which has recently come under significant criticism, is to look within these texts for subject matter with which one can then draw a one-to-one topical analogy to the contemporary problem at hand. And while this is a problem in academic Jewish ethics generally, it is a particular problem in Jewish sexual ethics.

If, however, we treat sex as not just "sex" but as a species of social intercourse, the range of texts available to the contemporary ethicist widens considerably. Now it is possible to engage potentially any text that has something to say about circumstances of social exchange in a conversation about sex and sexuality, because we understand that the text's observations about social exchange may be deeply relevant. In fact, as I demonstrate in chapter 5, because the activity of rabbinic textual interpretation is a social one, that activity itself may even become a source of moral reasoning patterns for the sexual ethicist. Furthermore, the insights we draw about ethics of relation-ship should, I argue, be applied in some form to our relationships with the scriptures upon which we draw. We ought not reduce our sexual and other-wise social partners to caricatures of either their worst or their best qualities, nor should we fully instrumentalize them. If we truly treat our scriptures *as* scriptures—which means, at least in part, that we understand them to have some sort of divinely given animation—we also need to apply these basic ethics of relationship to them.

Similarly, reading with attention to empirical pertinence also means at-tending to the particulars of what the relevant textual tradition says—or does not say!—on the subject rather than trading in abstract ideals about a tradi-tion's supposed "sex-positive" or "sex-negative" character. Textual traditions, much like human behavior, are multivalent, complex, and often frustrating, and they more than occasionally say things we as contemporary readers may not like. This does not mean that we must abandon our attempt to articulate from these texts rules by which we can live in our own particularity. It does mean, however, that we must do the work of wrestling with and accounting for what we find troubling in our texts.

Dialogue Partners: Crip Theory and Critical Disability Studies

I use crip theory and disability studies as theoretical frameworks for thinking about the moral meanings of everyday risks as embodied realities. Disability studies, as Aimi Hamraie succinctly puts it, developed as a stream of human-istic studies, one that centered a social model of disability that understood "disability [as] a socially and architecturally produced disadvantage [and] deemphasiz[ed] medical and scientific knowledge in favor of critical theory, qualitative data, and humanistic texts."[4] Crip theory simultaneously builds on and challenges this foundation, while drawing rhetorical and methodo-logical resources from queer theory. Crip theory, as Hamraie explains, "re-sists imperatives for normalization and assimilation [and] contribute[s] that disability is a valuable cultural identity, a source of knowledge, and a basis for relationality."[5]

Why these fields—and why risk? Risk is inherent in social interaction. This is because social interaction necessarily involves engaging with other agents, agents whose behavior one cannot fully control. Sex, clearly, is a form of social interaction of whose risks we are very well aware—in some cases, so much so to the point that we are inured to them. Sex carries concrete, physical risks of intimate partner violence, sexually transmitted infection (STI) transmission, and pregnancy, as well as less tangible yet equally real psychological and social risks.[6] Yet it is far from the only form of social interaction that carries such risks. Nonsexual social interactions also carry risks of contagion, violence, and social and psychological pain. Thus, in examining social risk more broadly, we can see the contiguities between sex and other forms of social intercourse. And, normatively speaking, the domain of risk—and the related domain of vulnerability—can help us understand the ways in which sexual interaction, attentively performed, can help shape us into more humane and attentive actors in *all* our social interaction.

The fields of crip theory and critical disability studies provide especially helpful discursive frameworks through which to understand how quotidian, nonsexual social interactions are fraught and risky in ways that we typically associate with sexual interactions. Disabled people regularly face a variety of obstacles that render the realities of day-to-day living risky and fraught, in ways that ought to be sharp and clear to all of us but which have been obscured and hidden, for the able-bodied, through compulsory able-bodiedness. I argue that the social riskiness that is often experienced quite sharply by disabled people elucidates something that is, in fact, profoundly true for all persons and all social interactions. Alison Kafer's apt parallel between compulsory able-bodiedness and compulsory heterosexuality is further true in that both systems—enabled, I argue, by the perception of sex as sui generis—seek to banish risk from "normal" or "healthy" interactions between "normal," "healthy" bodies and in doing so heap the risk onto interactions that fall outside those norms. But, of course, the risk is never banished; it is only veiled and ignored.

If the perception of sex as sui generis serves to occlude risk within certain approved spheres and multiplies it in ways that burden those acting outside approved spheres, one potential technology of repair is a recognition and a positive ethic of vulnerability. Here too, I argue, crip theory elucidates features of social interaction that are particularly apparent for disabled people but are, in the end, profoundly true for everyone. Crip voices and experiences classically expose the fiction of atomistic independence, highlighting instead the necessity for everyone of complex, interdependent webs of care and support. Recognizing this interdependence also means recognizing mutual vulnerability, for in our interaction with and interdependence on others, we necessarily reveal our weaknesses, hurts, and peculiarities. Choosing to reveal—and open up to damage—these things is the life-giving choice, because to avoid doing so is to close off the interaction and care we require to survive. At the same time, revealing particular vulnerabilities and needs becomes a way to ensure that any individual's identity and uniqueness is not lost within this interdependence.

Dialogue Partners: Empirical Accounts of Sexual Experience

Any adequate normative program must be closely and consistently attentive to the empirical realities of the phenomena it seeks to regulate. Put more simply: if we wish to regulate sex, we need to have an accurate and detailed account of what it is, how it works, and why we do it. This means attending to the empirical realities of actual human sexual behavior rather than to an abstract ideal of sexuality. Because I make normative claims about sex, basic interpretive care and attention to empirical pertinence require that I pay attention to how real people experience sex as an embodied phenomenon. Along these lines, I draw on sources like anthropologies of specific sexual communities (especially accounts of those organized around bondage/discipline/domination/submission/sadism/masochism, or BDSM), first-person accounts from sexual minorities as well as members of other marginalized communities, and psychological, sociological, and epidemiological studies of sexual behavior when I describe particular sexualities as sites and sources for moral reflection.

Why is this important, especially for a normative religious account of sexual ethics? Quite simply, without something like this, what ethicists talk about when they talk about sex is unlikely to have much in common with real sex lives. Lofty abstractions about divine union and fruitful mutuality look very nice on the printed page but have very little to do with the vast majority of people's actual experiences of sex. Sex is a real act that real, embodied people perform (even when sex is virtual, it's still performed by embodied actors), and if we want to have an adequate and practically helpful account of how people ought to interact sexually, we need to begin with an understanding of the ways people already interact sexually. This is not to commit the classic "is-ought" fallacy, in which we assume something ought to be a certain way because it already is a certain way. Rather, it is to say that practical sexual ethics should have concrete goals and that those goals will be much more humane and reachable if they are articulated in a way that accounts for actual people's behaviors, needs, and values. To simply say "don't do that" without giving a careful account of what people are doing and why they might be doing it is unlikely to meaningfully affect people's behavior. And to draw a picture of a sexual behavior or community we might go on to imagine as "deviant" without doing basic research into what might be happening is not only ineffective; it is dishonest and harmful.

Theoretical and Moral Commitments

I aim here to articulate a practical approach to Jewish sexual ethics that is queer, feminist, and sex positive. By "queer," I mean, broadly, that I understand the universe of potentially neutral or good sexual acts, preferences, and orientations to extend well beyond the limits set by conventional sexual mores; narrowly, I mean that my sexual ethics is particularly attentive to the needs and experiences of those within the queer (lesbian, gay, bisexual, transgender, intersex, and so on) community and is informed by my own experience as a queer person. By "queer," I also mean that my work is fundamentally informed by queer theory, in that it seeks to disrupt fixed, naturalized sexual and gender categories and hierarchies and that it begins with the premise that sex, sexuality, and gender are inextricably entangled with other social categories, structures, and identities.

By "feminist," I mean that I understand women as a class, in general and within Judaism in particular, to have been historically marginalized and disempowered relative to men as a class and to continue to be so in many ways. I see gender-based marginalization and disempowerment as morally wrong, and I seek, through my work here, to play a part in its continuing correction. I understand this correction as occurring through an ongoing exchange among core texts, traditions of reading, and ritual practices within Judaism and texts, traditions, and practices from both inside and outside Judaism that focus on naming, confronting, and repairing sex- and gender-based oppression. No tradition or community is either fully self-correcting or fully devoid of the internal resources for substantial self-correction, even if we were to assume the boundaries of such things were clear and impermeable.

By "sex positive," I mean that I take as a foundational premise the claim that sexual acts are, by themselves, morally neutral and that, all other things being equal, sexual fulfillment is a good that contributes in a substantial way to a person's flourishing. It is for this reason that I will refer to sexual "needs" as distinct from sexual "desires." I do not, in doing this, mean to say that one requires sex to live in the same way that one requires food, water, or oxygen, nor do I intend to erase the asexual community. What I do mean when I refer to "sexual needs" is that for people who are not asexual, sexual fulfillment is usually a very important component of their psychological and social well-being. One can surely live without sex, even if one is not asexual, as the experience of those whose religious vocations demand celibacy, for example, demonstrate. But it is often difficult and painful to do, especially outside the context of such a vocation, and the hunger for absent sexual fulfillment can be extraordinarily destructive.

Furthermore, the ability to pursue sexual fulfillment in a way that is coherent with one's identity is a form of self-expression that is integral to one's overall mental health. This is why Rabbi Steven Greenberg, in response to Orthodox puzzlement as to why Jewish law should give special treatment to sexually active gays and lesbians when it does not do so for people who violate other areas of halakhah, such as dietary law, retorts, "Nobody throws himself off a bridge because he or she is deprived of cheeseburgers."[7] While Greenberg is not referring to simple sexual fulfillment per se, he is claiming that the ability to live authentically as a sexual (or asexual) being is a fundamental and inextricable part of one's broader integrity and sense of self.

Learn from This: What Virtues Might We Cultivate When We Think Well with Sex and Texts?

How can thinking with texts in the ways I suggest throughout this book help us think better overall? What are the particular ways in which the study of sex is helpful in understanding other areas of social ethics? Do particular sexual *and* textual practices have the ability to teach specific virtues? What are the ways in which these practices cultivate virtue, and are there other specific social contexts in which the virtues cultivated by a particular sexual practice or a particular way of reading are especially useful? If Mira Balberg's analysis, which I discuss in chapter 4, is correct, purity and impurity functioned as paradigmatic sites for the cultivation of social and ritual virtue in the rabbinic world. Here in the contemporary world, sex and reading can function similarly as sites for the cultivation of social virtue.

While this book is far from comprehensive, the concepts and case studies I discuss here point to four particular virtues that can be cultivated by thinking with texts in the ways I suggest and by thinking about—and having, should it appeal!—good sex. These virtues have significant social value beyond either the textual or the sexual realm. These are *empirical justice, hermeneutic competency, wise risk management,* and *diverse interdependence.* Each is demonstrated and elucidated by the studies I undertake here, each corrects deeply rooted flaws in our collective thinking about sex, and each can be a valuable tool for building a more just society, sexually and otherwise.

<u>Empirical Justice</u>

Empirical justice is the normative corollary of the category of empirical pertinence, which I discuss above. Bluntly and crudely put, someone who exercises empirical justice is someone who *does the damn research.* More carefully put, to exercise empirical justice is to act and interpret in a way that recognizes the subjectivity and real testimony of one's interlocutor, whether that interlocutor is a text, a person, a practice, a community, an animal, an ecosystem, a ritual, a sensation. It is to acknowledge that one's interlocutors have, in the broadest sense of the term, reality that exists at least in part beyond one's own apprehension of them and to treat their communications regarding that reality as valid. Because all interactions are, at some level, acts of interpretation, empirical justice is a moral baseline for all social ethics.

Empirical justice can look very different depending on the context. If one is engaging with a body of text, empirical justice may mean working in careful dialogue with the text's narrative and poetic patterns and other formal features, its historical setting, its reception history, and its ongoing interpretive tradition. If one is engaging a person or a community, empirical justice means, at a minimum, taking their self-accounting seriously. If one is engaging with a set of practices—say, for an entirely random example, sexual practices—empirical justice means, at a minimum, learning what those practices entail and about the range of ways practitioners experience them. In all these cases, however, empirical justice begins with the understanding that one's interlocutor is more than one's metaphor, symbol, or thought experiment.

Where ancient texts and contemporary moral problems intersect, empirical justice requires readers to take the claims of both the text and the real people affected by the problem seriously. It requires neither reducing the text to a homily in support of one particular way of addressing the problem nor sacrificing the people whom the problem affects on the altar of textual solipsism. Empirical justice stands against textual apologia and textual disengagement alike. It stands against moral reductionism and against obfuscation of moral imperatives. It asks us to genuinely engage real complication, for it asks us to understand that real people live and die, suffer and flourish, within the details of a matter, but it warns us against introducing unnecessary complication or using complication as an excuse not to act.

Hermeneutic Competency

One uniting theme throughout the assortment of theoretical resources, rabbinic texts, and contemporary sexual case studies I treat throughout this book is that all social acts require some level of interpretation. We know that to read a text is to engage in acts of interpretation, and as I argue, how well and carefully we interpret our textual interlocutors has real consequences for the real people to whom those texts, in a variety of ways, matter. Similarly, to attend to one another's needs, vulnerabilities, desires, and imperfections— and to our own!—in a morally responsible way requires interpreting the ways we communicate with one another, verbally or otherwise.

Sexual interaction puts the moral centrality of interpretation into sharp relief. Are we able to interpret, for example, someone disclosing their HIV status as the wise and responsible act that it is, or do we interpret the information as a threat and mistreat its bearer? Can we effectively negotiate a sexual encounter and maintain a dialogue of ongoing consent throughout? Taking the time to establish a threshold of common communicative language prior to a sexual encounter and then paying sufficient attention to the ongoing communication that occurs throughout it is the difference between whether something is a morally acceptable sexual act or a reprehensible act of violence. Hermeneutic competency is, therefore, a moral imperative. And its stark centrality for sex demonstrates this in a way that should *highlight* its importance in other social situations. Negotiating consent is just as important, for example, in a medical setting as it is in a BDSM scene. Communicating one's health status—and responding with both interpersonal and material respect and charity to one who does—is as important in a whole range of interactions as it is with STIs.

What, precisely, does hermeneutic competency entail? Broadly speaking, it means treating any form of communication one receives, whether that be verbal, textual, bodily, or something else, with the care and consideration it deserves—and being deliberate about one's own communication in such a way that acknowledges its reception and interpretation by others. Part of developing hermeneutic competency is practicing the skills necessary to act with that care—skills that might include listening, reading, observing, and contextualizing. But even this development of skill is predicated on a basic respect for the subject of one's interpreting, for developing skills takes time and effort. Putting in that time and effort signals that one's subject is worth the work; failing to do so, and demonstrating that failure by interpreting one's subject badly or carelessly, by contrast, signals a fundamental lack of respect. In other words, the places we develop hermeneutic competency are fair indicators of our moral priorities.

There is no single technique, no one subject, no silver bullet that is The Answer to developing hermeneutic competency on a broad scale. Rather, different practices can help develop different aspects of hermeneutic competency and potentially address the risks and pitfalls of other practices. The study of Talmud, for example, inculcates a whole range of hermeneutic virtues (such as close reading and attention to detail, openness to multivalence, and collective, discursive study), but it on its own fails to prime its student to ask critical moral-hermeneutical questions like "Whose voice is missing?" Paired, however, with queer, feminist, womanist, and crip lenses, the study of Talmud can then prime one to ask precisely such questions, to perceive Talmud's moral-hermeneutical limits, and to look for sources and voices that speak from the perspectives that Talmud excludes and raise moral questions it cannot itself imagine.

Sex, similarly, can inculcate somatic-hermeneutical virtues. But it cannot do so in a vacuum. The ways we engage in sex condition the virtues and vices we develop through doing so. Having sex and thinking about sex with some of the same lenses that help students of Talmud develop socially responsible virtues—crip, queer, feminist, and womanist lenses—helps one develop a hermeneutic competency that, likewise, can ask, "Whose voice is missing? Who benefits? Who is being harmed? And how can I repair this?"

Wise Risk Management

Another theme common to all the texts I treat here is that they all deal with risk—its recognition, its acceptance, its moral qualities, its life-giving and community-building properties, and its wiser or more foolish management—in one form or another. Risk, as we shall see, has a great deal to do with sexual ethics; what we learn from thinking about sexual risk, in turn, has important implications for our social lives more generally.

Risk management has several aspects. This book draws out five notable ones, which I summarize here:

1. *Acceptance of risk.* The rabbinic texts I treat in this book all have risk of one kind or another as a constant and acknowledged interlocutor. Mishnaic purity discourse, which I discuss in chapter 4, assumes impurity to be default and ultimately unavoidable. Therefore, any rabbinic subject who enters any social sphere, no matter how assiduous their personal purity practice, knowingly risks contracting some form of impurity. The Oven of Akhnai narrative from Bavli Bava Metsia 59a–b, which I treat in chapter 5, spectacularly dramatizes the risks of engaging in communal study of and disputation over the interpretation of sacred text and shows its awareness of this risk by its setting in the midst of a discourse on the dangers of verbal wronging. The story of Rabbi Yoḥanan and Resh Lakish in Bava Metsia 84a, which I treat at the end of chapter 3, puts these dangers in more individual terms. The range of texts on execution that I discuss in chapter 5 show a powerful awareness of the political and moral risks of playing with power in the context of oppression at the hands of empire. And the story of Ḥaruta and R. Ḥiyya bar Ashi from Kidushin 81b, with which I conclude the book, poignantly showcases the risks of extreme askesis and stunted communication.

   Sexual interaction, too, is inherently risky. Persons who participate in sexual encounters place themselves in a position of physical and psychological vulnerability to their sexual partners. While these risks can be mitigated to a considerable degree, they can never be fully eliminated; indeed, part of what makes sexual interaction so appealing—and such an important site for moral and social development—is precisely the continuous presence of risk and vulnerability. To be ready for partnered sex is to accept that one is engaging in a risky activity and to be prepared to accept and manage any risks that do come to fruition.

Communities have a corresponding responsibility to describe and contextualize sexual risks accurately. It does little good if educators or community leaders play up the risks of one set of activities while downplaying the risks of others. Nor is it helpful if they fail to acknowledge that sexual actors balance multiple types of risks, frame sex as an outlandishly risky activity outside of specific and narrow standards, or frame sexual choices in terms of stark dichotomies of danger and safety. Rather, community leaders must understand sexual risks as existing within a broader web of social and physical risks and contextualize their messages accordingly.

2. *Self-awareness.* The Mishnah's major exhortation to individual moral actors regarding purity is one of constant self-awareness and self-examination. If impurity is ubiquitous, one who strives toward purity must begin by endeavoring to know their status at all times. Along these lines, all sexually active persons have, within reason, a duty of self-awareness. This refers most concretely to STI status; anyone who plans to engage in an activity that could transmit STIs should know what they may risk transmitting to their partners. But it also applies to other aspects of sexuality: someone who partici- pates in BDSM, for example, needs to be aware of their skill level at various activities, as well as having a reasonable awareness of the limit of what kind and how much play they can usually handle.

An important caveat here is that such awareness is always medi- ated by other factors. These factors may be primarily technical—for example, there is no reliable test for herpes in asymptomatic indi- viduals. They may be social, political, or economic—many people do not have reliable access to testing, or they may fear domestic or economic losses or violence if a positive test result becomes known. Some things may be genuinely unknowable in advance—psycho- logical triggers, for example, are notoriously unpredictable, and so someone may have no way of knowing that a new BDSM activity (or doing a familiar activity in a different setting) will be triggering until after the fact. Matters may even come down to prioritization— a genuinely monogamous long-term couple has no real need to test and retest themselves several years into their relationship. For these reasons, communities have a corresponding responsibility to make it convenient and acceptable for people to cultivate self-awareness. Sex education should emphasize pleasure, ongoing consent, regular STI testing, and the importance of masturbation both as self-care and as a means of discovering the particularities of one's own sexual response. STI testing should be free, easily accessible, confidential, and offered without shame.

There is also a broader responsibility for self-awareness, however: to be ready for partnered sex is, among other things, to have a certain basic knowledge of and comfort with one's own body and to have the beginnings of a reasonable idea of what one finds pleasurable, what one finds intolerable, and what one is and is not comfortable doing in a given moment. One is thereby better able to advocate for what they want in a sexual encounter. While one will likely discover the bulk of what one likes and dislikes sexually through experience with partnered sex, one can and should learn the basics of one's own sexual response through masturbation prior to engaging in partnered sex. Acquiring this basic knowledge is especially important for anyone who has been socialized as female, as this socialization often includes tacit or explicit cultural messages that women should not assert their sexual needs and that female sexual pleasure is unimportant or does not exist. Knowing that one is capable of experiencing sexual pleasure and knowing how to cause it is thus especially powerful.

3. *Mitigation of risk.* Just because risk is ubiquitous and actors have a duty to acknowledge and accept that, it doesn't follow that fatalism or apathy is acceptable. For example, the Mishnah, even though it treats impurity as commonplace, nevertheless scorns the *amei ha'arets* for their perceived failure to take available precautions and utilize mitigation strategies. The Oven of Akhnai, even as it recognizes the significant risks of debate in the bet midrash, is set within a discourse on the harms of verbal wronging, functioning within this context as an object lesson on the consequences of failing to observe sensible verbal precautions.

Likewise, while sexual interaction will never be—and often should not be!—risk-free, there is nevertheless much we can and should do to mitigate those risks. All sexually active persons—and, in some preventative cases, such as vaccines, all persons who may ever become sexually active—have a responsibility to utilize the best combination of protective measures for their particular situation. This includes discursive and hermeneutic skills like learning about and practicing ongoing enthusiastic consent, discussing preferences and negotiating scenes, and establishing safe words or similar structures. It also includes material interventions like seeking STI testing and treatment, getting immunized against such vaccine-preventable STIs as hepatitis B and cancer-causing strains of HPV, using barrier methods in any situation in which all parties are not reasonably sure of their STI status, and using PrEP for persons at high risk of contracting HIV. Communities, again, have corresponding responsibilities. Barrier methods should be widely available and free or low cost, and communities should actively work to encourage and destigmatize their use. Medical providers should actively encourage relevant vaccinations and other forms of prevention. Educators must actively work to dispel misinformation about these mitigation techniques. Communities, especially educators, must encourage and enable open, nonstigmatizing discussion of sexual health, sexual orientation, sexual pleasure, sexual diversity, and consent. Communities also have the responsibility to hold predators and other malevolent actors accountable.

4. *Discernment in weighing risks.* In almost any social situation, the operative question is not whether or not to take risks; rather, it is which risks one judges more worth taking than others. Discernment, which I discuss at length in chapter 3, is the virtue or skill necessary to make wise judgments about which risks to take to maintain individual and communal livability. Discernment means carefully observing, analyzing, weighing, and making careful judgments about information relevant to risks, both as they affect oneself and as they affect one's fellows. It also means admitting the limits of one's knowledge and understanding and knowing when to seek help. Along these lines, it also means recognizing that, all other things being equal, one is unlikely to be in a position to judge

others' discernment, because one is unlikely to have access to all the information that other person may be weighing. Therefore, charity and humility are bound up in discernment: to be humble and honest about the extent of one's own understanding and to be charitable about what may underlie others' decision-making is to be discerning about one's own and others' discernment.

Sexual discernment includes weighing the risks to oneself, one's partners, and one's extended sexual network of infection, injury, and social and emotional harm from encounters gone wrong alongside the sexual practices that are livable for them. It also includes weighing whether particular situations are worth potential risks that one perceives in them: Do I trust this particular person to top me? In this particular play party? If I feel uncomfortable about a particular partner, what am I basing that on? Is it worth voicing my discomfort to others? How might I weigh my communal obligations to warn people away from potential bad actors against my responsibility not to socially harm others without cause, particularly if I suspect my discomfort might be based in part on, say, socialized assumptions about race, class, and danger? Or, conversely, am I second-guessing my valid discomfort because gendered socialization has taught me to devalue my own judgment?

Sexual discernment also means not immediately assuming that someone who does not adhere to the same set of risk-management practices one has settled on for oneself therefore lacks discernment. Someone who has more sexual partners than one would think is appropriate might be reckless—or a livable sex life might, for them, require that amount of variety. Someone who hesitates to seek testing and treatment for STIs might be misinformed or irresponsible—or they might have very good reasons, such as a history of medical abuse, to avoid clinical settings.

Importantly, charitable discernment does not mean jettisoning communal norms. A community can and should hold that regular testing, treatment, vaccination, and prophylaxis of STIs is a prima facie duty incumbent on every sexually active person *and* at the same time acknowledge that some people may have good and valid reasons to avoid medical settings. It does not follow from this that the norm of testing, treatment, and prophylaxis should not be upheld; neither does it follow that people who have good reasons to avoid medical settings should be coerced into them regardless. Rather, the disjunction means that the community and the broader society have failed in their greater duty to create and foster conditions in which *everyone* is as safe and supported as possible in the course of carrying out their individual moral duties.

Diverse Interdependence

Sex is a matter of significant public and communal concern, and part of that concern is maintaining space for diversity of sexual expression. The parallel examples of the rabbinic bet midrash and present-day organized BDSM communities, which I treat at length in chapter 5, offer practical models for accomplishing this. The disputation that is at the center of the literary bet midrash requires internal difference to function, yet there are collective norms of behavior that govern and manage the discursive interactions between those differences in the interest of communal well-being. Similarly, organized BDSM is almost by definition a community structured around sexual difference, yet it too has communal norms that attempt to establish a baseline of communal well-being. Indeed, precisely because both communities are also organized around central, identity-defining risk activities, it is *especially* important for them to have robust communal norms and practices to manage those risks. Both the community's fundamental diversity and the risk-management practices the community generates help develop virtues that aid in risk management and mutual communal care and accountability, for different ways of being and different life experiences contribute a broader range of tools and knowledge that individuals and communities can deploy toward common goals of more livable, caring, accountable, and noncoercive societies. Diverse interdependence is therefore a communal virtue. It refers to those qualities and structures that allow a collective or community to create a whole that is greater than the sum of its parts and is capable of materially, socially, and spiritually supporting its members, while at the same time not merely allowing but fostering, valuing, and centering its members' diverse experiences, needs, perspectives, and ways of being.

One reason it is important to recognize, affirm, and accommodate different ways of being is that what is livable for one person may be unlivable or even deadly for another. It is important to be able to say that something is good for a given individual, for given communities, and for society at large *without* saying it is imperative for everyone to practice it. BDSM, when practiced responsibly, is good. The opportunity to practice it helps those who wish to make their lives livable, and the responsible practice of it develops virtues, like clear communication, negotiated ongoing consent, and general hermeneutic competency, that are good for *everyone* to develop and for society at large to encourage and foster. But it does not follow from this that everyone should practice BDSM. Indeed, for many people it may be unpleasant or even traumatic to practice it. We can recognize that BDSM is valuable in itself for some people, and a particularly good school for and source of virtues and norms that are good for most or all people, without claiming that all people therefore need to practice BDSM to recognize or benefit from what it has to offer. And the same, not incidentally, is true of Torah study.

One realm of difference that has particular moral import is that of power disparities, within which I include disparities of social, political, economic, and material wealth, power, privilege, and oppression. And it is especially critical for normative ethicists to be aware of the ways in which disparities of power affect people's relationships to moral norms. Take the example I treated above, in which some people may avoid STI testing and treatment because they have experienced medical abuse and can expect to experience it again. We can maintain that STI testing and treatment are still duties for everyone without condemning people who avoid it, because we recognize that the power disparities that affect them make the fulfillment of this duty more unlivable than other options. If there is a duty to seek a certain kind of care, and the care is abusive to at least some people who, as a result, avoid it, we can lay the dereliction of duty squarely at the feet of those institutions that made carrying out that duty unlivable or impossible.

Similar, then, to the recognition that something may be good without requiring that everyone do or aspire to do it, recognizing power disparities in a world short of *olam ha'ba*—the world to come—means recognizing that something can be a moral duty and that because of power disparities, it may be more difficult or even impossible for some people to carry that duty out. This does not mean that the duty is no longer incumbent on those people *or* that those people have failed in their duty—it means social duties are shared among individuals and the communities and societies they are part of and that society has failed in its duty to create morally livable conditions for all its members. Recognizing differences in power and the ways they affect one's ability to carry out moral duties is not moral individualism—rather, it is holding communities to their greater duties toward their members.

Background: Sex as Sui Generis and How It Got That Way

The argument that sex is a kind of social interaction—that it occurs as part of our social lives and shapes and is shaped by the same forces and structures that condition our other interactions—is familiar within the disciplines of queer and feminist studies, but it is seriously underutilized in religious ethics (womanist ethics being a notable exception) and especially in Jewish ethics.[8] What's more, its converse—that sex is its own country, a land of anarchy in the thrall of unreasonable, asocial, amoral passions—often goes unquestioned in both academic and lay discourse. There is, for example, no other form of social intercourse that we are exhorted to engage in with only one other person over the course of a lifetime. With the possible exception of consuming mind-altering substances, I can think of no other major social activity from which entire classes of people are, under normal circumstances, enjoined to abstain in perpetuity on account of its attendant risks. Or consider the prejudice against sex work: there is something many of us, feminist thinkers very much included, find appalling about exchanging sex for money. This is despite the fact that there are a number of other professions whose basis is the exchange of either bodily services or social intimacy for money: Martha Nussbaum systematically compares sex work with a number of other occupations—including professor of philosophy—along these very lines.[9] Two professions she does not treat but which would also fit the analysis are that of professional athlete and clergyperson.[10] Similarly, there are any number of industries with serious worker exploitation and human trafficking problems, notably agriculture and construction; sex work is hardly unique in this respect, either.[11]

How did things get this way? It is not possible to pinpoint a specific moment in Western history and say, "There, *that* is when sex became sui generis!" Various historical trends have, however, contributed, in one way or another, to the treatment of sex as such. Some of these trends are philosophical and theological, while others are based more tangibly in, say, monastic or scientific practices. Generally speaking, many of these trends find their roots in ancient and early Christian and, to a lesser extent, Jewish thought about sex and sexuality. In early Christianity in particular, fornication began to emerge as a singular sin that was related to—in fact, foundational to—but distinct from other disordered appetites. While the early Stoics may have had an understanding of sexuality precisely as a communal phenomenon, a social interaction that could be rational and through whose wise practice one could develop virtues, by the time of the later Stoics, especially the Roman Stoics, sexual desire "is nothing more than the passion that it was in popular Greek thought."[12] Pythagoreanism contributed the view, adopted in later Christian thought as "procreationism," that "sexual relations should be practiced strictly in a temperate and deliberately reproductive way, and solely within marriage."[13] From the Hebrew Bible, we get the recurring motif, illustrated perhaps most vividly in the prophetic literature, of sexual transgression as a metonym for communal discord and as a metaphor for idolatry and communal transgression of divine law.[14] Paul, drawing on all these traditions, distinguishes lust from other appetites and passions, "set[ting] sexual fornication in a class of danger by itself because of the body with which he associates the violation. On his view the body is the collective of Christians as corporate bride . . . [who] need to uphold the bride's chastity through their own sexual bodies."[15]

Thus the idea that sex has distinct and often baneful significance became integral to its treatment in Western culture.[16] This idea of sex as a separate and private category was reified by the reframing of sex as a category of scientific study beginning in the Enlightenment and continuing into the nineteenth and twentieth centuries. In this period, even as sexual deviance was framed as a broader social problem, the taxonomization and naturalization of sexual difference and the insistence that "proper" sexual conduct belonged in the private sphere served to reify the "givenness" of accepted sexual practices, while sequestering actual sexual interaction behind closed doors and away from other forms of social intercourse.[17] And this public/private dichotomy continues even to today: even as our public discourse is saturated with and sensationalized by sexual imagery, actual sexual praxes and discourses continue to be privatized and barred from "respectable" public spaces.

Along these lines, it is important to note that the treatment of sex as sui generis is not usually absolute, either in theory or in practice. A thinker may have a philosophical understanding of sex as socially integrated while nevertheless normatively treating it as though it were quite distinct from other social phenomena. Others might treat sex, both normatively and descriptively, as socially integrated in some areas but not in others. This ambiguity, too, has roots in antiquity: as Kathy L. Gaca notes, the early Stoics, especially Zeno and Chrysippus, understood well-ordered eros as a form of rational discourse and a means of developing and sustaining friendships as befits humanity's naturally gregarious character. However, mixing sex with the social activity of commerce crossed a line for these thinkers—the commercial exchange of sex, even if fully consensual, was a disordered manifestation of eros.[18]

None of this is to say that there are not specific ways in which we habitually connect sex to other parts of our social lives. On the contrary: sexual virtue is *constantly* linked to other social virtues, and sexual deviance is figured as singularly destructive to the bedrock of our social institutions. Yet even in its linkage *to* other forms of sociality, sex is held curiously apart: it becomes metonymic for social function or dysfunction, or, even more intensely, it becomes the singular foundation for that function or dysfunction.

Regardless of how it came to be and whether or not it is explicitly acknowledged, the consequences for practical ethics, especially Jewish ethics, of treating sex as a sui generis category, are twofold: First, it allows ethicists to treat sex in far stricter terms than they otherwise would and to treat sexual problems, especially where power dynamics are concerned, in partial or total isolation from the wide range of social forces that influence them or the actual lives of the people who experience them. Second, it limits ethicists to a narrow range of classical source texts whose subject matter is explicitly sexual. This, in turn, foreshortens the range of traditionally grounded patterns with which the ethicist can think through practical questions of sex and sexuality. In short, the consequences of this categorization line up rather well indeed with the two major components of the problems I identified at the beginning of this section with academic Jewish sexual ethics as it stands today. This book, then, begins to address these components by taking sex's social character seriously.

Plan of the Book

This book is divided into two parts. Part I builds a hermeneutical and theoretical scaffold for my work. Part II uses that scaffolding to examine two case studies, which I treat as specific applications of my broader argument. Here, I apply the broader claims I make in part I, drawing out specific ways that these claims can apply to questions of risk management and sociosexual formation.

Chapter 1 lays out my hermeneutic methodology and, in doing so, details the book's parameters as a work of *Jewish* thought. It grounds my argument in Jewish text and offers a new hermeneutical approach to doing contemporary ethics with classical rabbinic texts. Here, I argue that my claim, that sex is not sui generis but is rather a species of social intercourse, is not only practically liberatory: it is hermeneutically liberatory as well. As I note above, contemporary Jewish practical ethics tends to limit itself to rabbinic material whose surface-level subject matter appears to align with the contemporary problem under discussion; this tendency is particularly egregious in Jewish sexual ethics. Such hermeneutic praxis leads to a kind of simplistic proof texting in which the text or texts say what the tradition "thinks" about the contemporary problem; the ethicist must then either defend "the tradition's viewpoint" or explain why rejecting it is warranted. This sort of proof texting tends to greatly oversimplify the dynamics in a particular text and collapse context such that the phenomenon under discussion in the text is assumed to be more or less the same thing as the contemporary problem.

If, however, we understand sex as a species of social interaction, it is far easier to see how texts whose subject matter is not explicitly sexual can nevertheless offer contemporary ethicists practical guidance on questions of sexuality. Other areas of Jewish ethics already make similar moves; a text about a rabbi's martyrdom at the hands of Rome, for example, seems to have little to do with present-day medicine, and yet the martyrdom of Rabbi Ḥanina as told in Bavli Avodah Zarah 18a has become a key text with which Jewish bioethicists think about end-of-life decision-making. Any text about some aspect of social interaction may prove helpful. Indeed, because the rabbis understood sex as a fundamentally different sort of thing than most of us do today, it may often be the case that texts that are not explicitly sexual are *more* useful for contemporary sexual ethics than are explicitly sexual ones.

The first section of this chapter explores the reasons why contemporary ethicists should look past simple subject matter when using rabbinic texts. I argue that most of the explicitly sexual material in rabbinic texts shows that sex almost always functions for the rabbis in one of three ways: as a tool for the demarcation and enforcement of social and economic boundaries, as an arena for the performance of sagely virtue and rabbinic authority, or as a tool for solving a particularly thorny interpretive problem. More broadly, I argue, in concurrence with a number of recent studies of rabbinics, that rabbinic texts are not primarily about any given practical concern. Instead, rabbinic texts are primarily about rabbinic interpretive methods, rabbinic character, and rabbinic authority. These texts are profoundly self-focused and self-referential; as a consequence, we as readers should be extremely careful about assuming anything about their subject matter without considering what that subject matter meant in the rabbinic textual and intellectual world.

The second section of this chapter advances an alternative methodology for deriving meaningful contemporary content from rabbinic subject matter. Rather than focusing on decontextualized subject matter, I argue that it is more helpful to examine how particular social phenomena function within the rabbinic world and then compare aspects of this to the ways the contemporary problem functions. Thus, for example, ritual impurity functions in the rabbinic world as an unavoidable socially transmitted contagion. While there is no literal analogue to ritual impurity in the contemporary world, there are several types of unavoidable socially transmitted contagion—including sexually transmitted infections—that function quite similarly to the ways ritual impurity functions in the rabbinic world.

The final section of the chapter attempts to distill the beginnings of an ethics of interpretation from the work done in the previous sections. For, if it is a text-historical truth about rabbinic texts that they are fundamentally about the rabbis and their world, it is a religious truth, at least for those to whom rabbinic texts are sacred texts, that these texts have a weight, a moral standing, and an ineluctably interactive character all their own. Such character means that these texts merit being treated by their interpreters in specific ways. I argue that the fundamental grounding of such treatment mirrors the mutual vulnerability that, as I go on to argue, both good sex and crip theory also model for us: a mutual willingness to be encountered, touched, changed, and potentially hurt by the other, as well as a refusal to shy away from potentially changing the other oneself. At the same time, one must also be willing to encounter the other honestly—as that other is, in their full context, rather than as what one wishes the other to be.

While chapter 1 is a methodological and hermeneutical scaffold for my text work, chapter 2 is a theoretical scaffold for my thought about sex as a social phenomenon. Here, I give a detailed account of sexual interaction as a form of social intercourse. I examine the goods of pleasure and diversity as they function in relation to sex and compare this to the functions of pleasure as it relates to the social experiences of eating and drinking, and of diversity as it relates to the lived social experiences of disabled (and especially neurodivergent) people. First, I offer an account of pleasure, including bodily pleasure, as fundamentally social. While the physiology of pleasure may be a largely individual phenomenon, the fact remains that a significant part of our basic social infrastructure is formed around the communal production and experience of bodily and psychological pleasures. One of the critical ways in which we form communal bonds, in other words, is by feeling good together. I develop this account of pleasure as a socially enmeshed and formative category through an extended comparison with the social functions of the bodily pleasures we derive from eating and drinking. I also flag some of the potential discontents of "community" as a normative category that I address later in this chapter, as well as in chapter 5.

I then argue, continuing my analogy to the pleasures of eating and drinking, and building on Alasdair McIntyre's concept of the "polymorphous character of pleasure," that pleasure is an idiosyncratic, protean, and diverse phenomenon.[19] Further, I argue, this diversity is morally valuable, both individually and collectively, in its own right, and communities should accommodate and, indeed, foster such. Drawing on the neurodiversity paradigm, which argues that neurological differences like autism and ADHD are valuable ways of perceiving and being in the world in their own right, I argue that divergent ways of experiencing pleasure (which, like neurodivergences, are in one important sense differences of *social perception*) are valuable as specific generators of interpersonal duties and as sources of a rich, varied, and sometimes unexpected range of virtues and moral disciplines. I also introduce crip theory as an analytic framework for thinking about divergence, using the link that discipline draws between compulsory heterosexuality and compulsory able-bodiedness both to underscore the worth of bodies and ways of being that have been labeled "deviant" and to prefigure the discussion of deviance and risk in the next section. Queerness and disability are both types of physical and social deviance, the particulars of which are often constructed in intimate relation to forms of risk that become either inextricable from or fundamentally inimical to those ways of being.

Chapter 3 considers risk as a moral category. Contrary to accounts that move to restrict sexual expression on the grounds of sex's putatively singular risks, I argue that *all* forms of social interaction are inherently risky and that many commonplace forms of it carry similar physical and socioemotional risks to those we primarily associate with sex. Continuing along the previous chapter's two comparative axes, I discuss the commonplace risks of physical injury and infectious disease, as well as the psychosocial risks of humiliation and rejection that come with cooking, eating, and drinking. Using crip theory—and I draw in particular on the work of Robert McRuer, Carrie Sandhal, and Alison Kafer—as a framework from which to think through social risk and its moral value, I note that the linked systems of compulsory heterosexual and compulsory able-bodiedness paint a picture of an ideal (yet impossible) way of being that is free from risk.[20] Both systems—enabled, I argue, by the perception of sex as sui generis—seek to banish risk from "normal" or "healthy" interactions between "normal," "healthy" bodies and in doing so heap the risk onto interactions that fall outside those norms. But, of course, the risk is never banished; it is only veiled and ignored. Thus both crip and queer experience testify to the impossibility of this picture. I discuss the ways these parallel risks of everyday nonsexual interaction are heightened for disabled people and hold up the techniques disabled people regularly use to acknowledge and manage these risks as virtues all of us, regardless of ability or impairment, would do well to cultivate throughout our social lives, sexual and otherwise.

At the end of the chapter, I introduce two concepts for thinking with and about risk: *livability* and *discernment*. Livability—by which I mean a state of dynamic balance among one's needs and desires, the needs and desires of one's individual social interlocutors, and the basic structures of one's community, such that everyone may flourish and no one experiences unbearable hardship—is a way of describing the goal of wise risk management. Discernment—by which I mean the capacity to observe, balance, and carefully judge information about risks and goods as they may affect oneself and others—is a keystone virtue that enables wise risk management. Finally, as a transition between the conceptual chapters in part I and the case studies in part II, I offer a brief reading of the story, in Babylonian Talmud (Bavli) Bava Metsia 84a, of Rabbi Yoḥanan and Resh Laḳish, through the lens of social risk. Their ultimately tragic story, I argue, serves as a poignant study both of the deep and significant risks of intimate social interaction and of the life-giving character of those very risks.

Chapter 4 is the first of two case studies that form part II of the book. In this chapter, through a close reading of selected passages from Mishnah Zavim, I draw a parallel between STIs and mishnaic ritual impurity. Drawing on Balberg's account of ritual impurity in the Mishnah, I argue that ritual impurity—a metaphysical condition that is incompatible with contact with the sancta and is spread by direct and indirect physical contact—is figured as an unavoidable consequence of routine forms of social interaction, forms that are in and of themselves desirable. [21] I do this by way of central claims, two of which emerge through Balberg's broader analysis and two of which emerge from my reading of Zavim. First, ritual impurity, which travels through shifting webs of contagion, is a ubiquitous, unavoidable presence in the tannaitic social world. Second, because of this ubiquity, the moral focus of impurity discourse is not on the impurity itself nor on the actions that might transmit it but rather on the process of managing and ameliorating the transmission of impurity. Third, this world in which impurity is unavoidable is also one in which intimate human interaction—which is both a path of transmission for impurity and, often, desirable in and of itself—is also unavoidable. Finally, because of all these factors, the ethical management of impurity is characterized by a multifactorial process of discussion, diagnosis, and response.

I bridge this mishnaic analysis to contemporary problems of sex and public health by arguing that STIs are also forms of socially transmitted contagion that are ultimately unavoidable consequences of desirable and routine forms of social interaction. The mishnaic model of extensive discussion and matter-of-fact management and amelioration is therefore a helpful model for responding to STIs and for a practical ethics of sex and public health more generally. In this section, I draw out this functional parallel by rereading the texts from Zavim onto contemporary STI management problems, thereby highlighting specific ways in which the phenomena of mishnaic impurity and STIs are descriptively similar and laying out a normative agenda for STI management that is rooted in mishnaic management strategies.

Chapter 5's case study draws a parallel between organized BDSM practice and the activity of rabbinic text interpretation. Through a close reading of the classic Oven of Akhnai narrative in Bavli Bava Metsia 59a–b, I argue, building on Jeffrey Rubenstein's classic accounts of rabbinic verbal violence and Jonathan Schofer's treatment of the moral and metaphysical risks of engaging with and interpreting scripture, that the activity of interpretation is figured within rabbinic text as a risky activity with potential social, psychological, theological, and even physical consequences.[22] The activity of text interpretation is a risky yet, at the same time, strongly desired activity—as well as being an activity that becomes constitutive of rabbinic identity. The community of the bet midrash is formed around this activity and develops rules and structures of communal authority designed to contain and manage the risks inherent in it.

Such a description also applies to organized BDSM communities. Drawing on Staci Newmahr's and Margot Weiss's anthropological accounts, as well as firsthand accounts and educational essays from BDSM practitioners, I show that here, too, a community is formed around a desired, risky activity, one that is often significantly constitutive of its members' identities. And here, too, the community exists in large part to regulate and manage the acknowledged risk, creating rules, technologies, and scripts designed to force explicit confrontation of and engagement with that risk, as well as looking out for bad actors that elevate risks beyond an acceptable level. Thus, both the bet midrash, or study house, of classical rabbinic text and the contemporary organized BDSM dungeon are examples of what I call "risk-conditioned communities."

These communities, I argue, model social virtues in three ways: First, they assume that disciplines practiced in and for a specific community have moral value well beyond that context. Second, they model the development of broader virtues through the practice and refinement of specific technical skills. Of particular note here is both communities' emphasis on *hermeneutic* skills: those of text interpretation and disputation in the rabbis' case and those of negotiating questions of ongoing consent and physical and psychological comfort and safety in the BDSM practitioners' case. Finally, both communities—especially the BDSM community—build communal bonds and cultivate specific shared virtues and skills *without* flattening, eliding, or eliminating difference and diversity within that community. Organized BDSM in particular, as a community by definition organized *on the basis of* sexual difference, can offer a model of community that affirms and fosters the kind of difference and diversity whose value I established in chapter 2. Here, I argue, are the beginnings of a model of communal investment in sexual well-being: one in which sex is a public matter but in which variation, diversity, and realistic risk assessment are acknowledged and accepted. In each case, the community acknowledges, accommodates, and manages a wide variety of individual expression within its regulatory structures.

If the bet midrash and the dungeon share morally salutary features, however, they also share discontents. Drawing on Margot Weiss's *Techniques of Pleasure: BDSM and the Circuits of Sexuality*—an anthropology of organized BDSM in the San Francisco Bay Area—and Beth Berkowitz's analysis of execution rituals in tannaitic (early rabbinic) literature (mainly, Mishnah Sanhedrin), I argue that rabbinic discourse and organized BDSM share a similarly complex and troubled relationship of resistance, reappropriation, and reproduction—a kind of relationship Weiss calls a "circuit"—with the power structures as whose antitheses they style themselves. Just as organized BDSM reproduces neoliberal hierarchies (for example, of socioeconomic class, given the often staggering monetary and time investment in equipment and classes that many communities have come to expect) and rigid sexual categories (cordoning off "vanilla" praxis from that which it deems sufficiently "queer"), so too did the rituals of execution found in rabbinic texts reproduce Roman technologies and social dynamics of execution.

However, where much organized BDSM maintains, according to Weiss, a rhetoric of separation from those broader social dynamics through its appeal to the theatrical, staged character of its practice, the rabbinic texts display a keen awareness of their troubled relationship with Roman themes and power structures. The rabbis, for all their discontents, know very well that play is more than "just" play and that text is more than "just" text, and they consciously engage these troubled relationships as a form of subversion and resistance, in a way that Berkowitz compares to the postcolonial theorist James Scott's concept of the "hidden transcript."[23] In this, they—along with multiply marginalized players within the BDSM scene, such as the Black women players analyzed by Ariane Cruz and Amber Jamilla Musser and disabled players, like the performance artist Bob Flanagan—offer to those of us (all of us) enmeshed in such circuits the beginnings of a technology of acknowledgment and repair.[24]

In the book's conclusion, I argue that the contiguity between sex and other forms of social interaction, as elucidated throughout, has implications beyond sexual ethics. Indeed, because of sex's status on the one hand as a species of social interaction, and because of the particular anxieties its especially obvious fleshliness arouses on the other, sex is a particularly important area of study for *all* social ethicists. Because sex tends to intensify the dynamics found in other types of social interaction, studying sex helps us see more clearly the most important aspects of a number of broader questions in social ethics. Feminist and womanist ethicists have already discovered this fact, but their insights remain due for broader uptake across the discipline of ethics. Virtue ethicists, for example, can find in sexual practices potential sites for social self-formation; partnered sex can train moral actors in practices of attentiveness, care, and humane response to vulnerability. And, as I note at length in chapter 5, communitarian ethicists can look to particular sexual subcultures, such as BDSM groups, for both positive and negative examples of how to practice communal care, accountability, and formation of common norms and narratives.

On Writing about Social Risk in a Pandemic

When I began to work on this project, I could not have anticipated that my claims about the risky character of all kinds of day-to-day social interaction would be demonstrated by the COVID-19 pandemic with devastating clarity. Nor, perhaps foolishly, did I anticipate that the reality of ever-present social risk would be so thoroughly weaponized against life-saving public health measures as it has been. Yet as I prepared the final revision of this manuscript in the summer of 2021, and *still*, as I prepare the final copy edit in the summer of 2022, that is where we are. Therefore, it seems to me that some moral clarification is in order.

What I argue throughout this book—that even the most quotidian, mundane, G-rated sorts of social interactions carry risks that are contiguous with those of sex, that daily life involves constant negotiation and management of these risks, and that the existence of these risks does not and ought not negate the benefits of our daily social interactions—the COVID-19 pandemic has driven home repeatedly and forcefully. Many of us have, in the wake of the pandemic's attendant lockdowns, come to realize intimately and painfully how life-giving those activities that COVID-19 rendered life-*threatening* truly are for us. We have been forced to grapple with the necessity of weighing our mental, social, and economic well-being against the real and immediate risk of contracting and spreading a pathogen that can sicken, disable, and kill us and those we love and has caused and continues to cause suffering, death, and socioeconomic calamity on a global scale.

However, there are also some significant ways in which the pandemic warrants special consideration, both in terms of the ways it is contiguous with my overarching arguments here and the ways it departs from them. First, the account I just gave in the previous paragraph is at best incomplete. The "we" in that paragraph figures the default pre-COVID experience as nondisabled, white, cis, male, heterosexual, and economically secure. People who fall outside that charmed circle (to apply Gayle Rubin's terminology to a different context) have already been forced to grapple with the riskiness of everyday activities and to choose among necessities on a regular and un-relenting basis.[25] To say COVID-19 has newly forced "us" to confront these things is to say that the experiences of those outside this charmed circle are practically and morally insignificant and, indeed, to say that they lack a degree of moral standing.

At the same time, COVID-19 puts those of us who dwell outside that charmed circle at even more acute risk. This means that for those within the circle to decide that the value of everyday activities they were used to prepandemic outweigh the value of pandemic restrictions is to decide that the value of their activities also outweighs the pleasure, well-being, and lives of those outside it. Being cavalier about COVID-related risks has a dispro-portionately large impact on whether disabled and chronically ill people, for example, get to exist in public at all. What's more, the increased restrictions on daily activities during COVID aren't meant to be constants; they're meant to arrest an acute and heightened risk so that ultimately *no one* must shoulder undue and unnecessary burdens of social risk. The laxer people within the circle are about vaccination, masking, social distancing, and other contain-ment measures, the longer those outside the circle will have to maintain the strictest possible measures across all aspects of their lives just to stay alive.

So yes, lockdowns, distancing, masking, and other social interventions are genuinely hard and bear their own real and significant risks and harms. It is also *indisputably* the case that the oppressive structures in which we are all already entangled shift the worst burdens of those interventions onto those who were already shouldering undue hardship and harm. For them, what I argue in this book *indeed* has very significant continuity with the current situation, and those of us with relatively more social power *should* be asking why some people's mental and social well-being has become even more unimportant. Those of us who already bear these burdens have exercised supererogatory empirical justice, hermeneutic competency, wise risk management, and diverse interdependence and continue to do so, and the proper response is not to condemn but to materially support.

For those of us, however, who are only now confronting this need to weigh such well-being against the risks of direct and acute physical harm to themselves and others, to decide to ignore the most basic of public health safeguards because "life is risky" doesn't display *any* of these virtues. It only displays callous indifference and unwillingness to take on even a slight, temporarily higher risk burden for the sake of their fellows.

For shame.

PART I

Groundings

1. TEXTUAL INTERCOURSE

Grounding Sexual Ethics in Jewish Sources

I CLAIM THROUGHOUT THAT this book is a Jewish argument about social ethics, and so it stands to reason that I must engage with some Jewish
sources, whether those sources be textual, ritual, or ethnographic in nature.
Here, my main Jewish sources are textual ones: like most of my colleagues
and predecessors in the field of applied Jewish ethics, I ground my reasoning
in the vast and sprawling canon of classical rabbinic text.[1]

However, I deploy these texts in different ways than most of my predecessors in this field have. As I discuss in detail below, I believe that simply applying the surface meaning of rabbinic texts' subject matter to superficially
similar contemporary problems too often yields an ethics that is theoretically
impoverished, hermeneutically questionable, and insufficiently attentive to
the empirical realities of the situations it seeks to address. Ethicists should
instead deploy texts in ways that are attentive to the nuances both of their
subject matter and of their formal structure: to the power dynamics that
unfold in them, to the patterns of thought and interlocution of their arguments, to the sweeps and zigzags of their narrative arcs, and to the social and
theological intricacies they describe and imagine.

This chapter explicates the method of text reading I use throughout the
book. It also makes the case that, just as substantially dissolving what I argue
is an artificial boundary between sex and the rest of sociality helps to make us
better thinkers and actors, we can benefit similarly by dissolving the boundaries that limit classical Jewish texts to readings that foreground revelation
or piety. In what follows, I describe my own emergent ethical hermeneutic

process. In the first section, I explain why I think it is insufficient to "do" practical Jewish ethics by drawing simple one-to-one correspondence between a contemporary problem and the immediate subject matter of a given text. In the second section, I describe an alternative hermeneutic (which I hope will be one of many possibilities) that interrogates the social functions of a text's subject matter within its own textual world and then seeks out functional parallels in contemporary problems. Finally, in the third section, I argue that to practice a more nuanced hermeneutic methodology, such as the one I have offered, conditions the practitioner as a social and moral actor in particular and important ways—that, in other words, the hermeneutical interaction with text is, like sex, a particular form of social intercourse with its own particular yet more broadly connected virtues.

Looking beyond Simple Subject Matter

One critical task for the Jewish ethicist who wishes to read classical texts in ways that do not center piety or revelation is to critically interrogate regnant apologetic readings of those texts. For the sexual ethicist, one of these regnant claims looms larger than others—namely, that "the Jewish tradition," and specifically classical rabbinic texts, are notably "sex positive," especially compared to regnant Christian accounts of sex and sexuality. Yet this claim that the Jewish tradition (if one can even refer to it in the singular) is either "sex positive" or "sex negative" is at best a simplistic account of the corpus's engagement with sexual subject matter. It also forecloses critical engagement with explicitly sexual texts and discourages sexual ethicists' attention to other potentially generative texts whose subject matter is not explicitly sexual. Different streams of tradition, at different points in history, demonstrate different trends in their approach to sex and sexuality.[2] To recover a nuanced and workable sexual ethic from Jewish tradition requires more than simply identifying and mapping these trends. Such a recovery requires a different hermeneutical approach, one that is attentive to the complex character of the various trends within Jewish traditions, of the equally complex character of its contemporary ethical subject, and of the specific claims and needs of the activity of articulating normative ethics. As such, I argue, explicitly sexual texts may not prove to be our best resources for present-day sexual ethics. However, other texts, as I discuss in the next section of this chapter, may prove far more fruitful and thought-provoking.

How Jewish Normative Ethics Tends to Use Rabbinic Text

As Emily Filler has noted, extensive reference to and use of classical rabbinic sources is almost omnipresent in Jewish ethics.[3] Yet too often, these texts are used as though they contain simple one-to-one analogs to the problems with which contemporary ethicists grapple. As the ethicist Louis Newman, who provides perhaps the most extensive internal critique of what we might call the "proof texting" of rabbinic sources by contemporary Jewish ethicists, puts it, "Virtually all exegetes employ a model of textual interpretation which assumes first, that texts themselves contain some single determinate meaning and second, that the exegete's role is to extract this meaning from the text and apply it to contemporary problems."[4] Such assumptions, Newman insists, are "questionable, if not altogether untenable."[5] Similarly, within the discipline of rabbinics, Elizabeth Shanks Alexander, Beth Berkowitz, Mira Balberg, and Charlotte Fonrobert, among others, have all argued convincingly that it is problematic to try to straightforwardly deploy the content of rabbinic texts in the service of contemporary ethical-normative claims. To do so, they note, is to miss a defining characteristic of rabbinic text: it is primarily about the rabbis and their world.

Beth Berkowitz offers a particularly strong exposition of this problem. In *Execution and Invention: Death Penalty Discourse in Early Rabbinic and Christian Cultures*, Berkowitz examines the modern reception history of rabbinic texts that deal with the topic of capital punishment. American Jewish writers, according to Berkowitz, "want to know: What is the traditional Jewish perspective on capital punishment?"[6] She identifies a tradition, beginning in the late nineteenth century, of reading Talmudic texts on criminal justice as models of humanitarianism. Using a passage from Mishnah Makot 1:10—"R. Ṭarfon and R. Akiva declare that, had they been members of the Sanhedrin, a sentence of death would never have been passed"—as his central proof text, an obscure rabbi and lawyer by the name of Samuel Mendelsohn "goes so far as to say that the Talmud's ethics were not only progressive by modern standards, but even more progressive than modern standards."[7] This proof text continues to appear in abolitionist writings throughout the twentieth century, usually omitting, as Mendelsohn did, the very next phrase: "Rabbi Shimon ben Gamliel said, they would thereby have increased bloodshed in Israel." There is also a countertradition, which Berkowitz grounds in mid-twentieth-century Israeli thought but which is also evident in American thought, with such writers as Walter Jacob and David Novak arguing that "the Rabbis were fundamentally in favor of the death penalty despite several statements to the contrary."[8]

Such writers—both those who are in favor of capital punishment and those who are against it—Berkowitz argues, miss the actual trees for an impressionist painting of a forest. First, each side is likely to underrepresent texts that complicate their case; abolitionist readers, for example, tend to ignore the final clause of M. Makot 1:10, while readers who advocate for capital punishment similarly tend to minimize texts that express opposition not just to frequent executions but to any executions at all. Even where writers represent this intrarabbinic debate more fairly, they tend to focus largely on the texts about *whether* capital punishment should occur, at the expense of those texts that describe the rabbinic rituals of execution themselves. Berkowitz writes, "Looking at what happens *after* conviction . . . makes it possible to move beyond either/or thinking about rabbinic criminal execution [to] explore the rabbinic death penalty as a social, political, and religious practice."[9] Such exploration, she argues, yields the conclusion that rituals of execution are ultimately about rabbinic discourses of power and the power of rabbinic discourse, "not just about criminals and courts but about the power of the Rabbis to redeem any Jew."[10]

Berkowitz's observations ring true for more than just death penalty discourse. Contemporary Jewish ethicists regularly characterize rabbinic discourse as being affirming of sex and sexuality. Thus, for example, Eliott Dorff cites Mishnah Ketubot 5:6, which specifies how often a man in a given profession owes his wife sex, and M. Ketubot 5:7, which stipulates that a wife who withholds sex from her husband shall have her *ketubah* money docked, as proof that the rabbis, and Jewish values generally, support an active and mutual marital sex life. As compared to the views of "other societies" in the ancient, medieval, and modern worlds, which ascribe sexual desire to men alone,[11] Dorff argues that these texts, among others, demonstrate that "the Torah, and the Rabbis who later interpret it, [recognize] the couple's mutual desires."[12] Along similar lines, he cites Bavli Eruvin 100b, which features an extended discussion of whether it is acceptable for a husband to force his wife to have sex with him and whether it is proper for a wife to demand sex from her husband, and Bavli Yevamot 62b, which discusses certain conditions under which a wife's desire for her husband may be especially strong, as evidence that "the Jewish tradition . . . instructs men to be sensitive to their wives' intimations of the desire for sex and to satisfy that need whenever possible."[13]

It is inarguable that many of these texts have, in fact, served as the bases for a great deal of normative sexual halakhah. But the claims Dorff is making here go beyond halakhah and into the realm of values. Beyond ruling, in his capacity as a posek, that Jewish law mandates a certain program of sexual conduct for husbands and wives, Dorff is claiming that the Jewish tradition values mutual desire within marital sex and that this value comes from the same value as demonstrated in classical rabbinic text.

It is this latter claim that I consider dubious, for this chapter's closer look at the texts that specifically engage sexuality reveals that within these texts, discourse on sex has more to do with establishing social, familial, and religious boundaries—and the rabbis' authority to define them—as well as setting the stage for stories of exemplary sagely conduct than it does with sex for its own sake. The claim that rabbinic text is somehow sexually affirming is not only debatable at best; it is beside the point, because the text is not primarily about sex or sexuality. Rabbinic text is about rabbinic text, rabbinic character, and rabbinic authority; it is about sex and sexuality mainly inasmuch as those topics provide interesting cases or ways to think through a textual issue—and to affirm rabbinic claims of authority.

Explicitly Sexual Texts and What Is and Isn't Going On in Them

At first glance, it certainly appears as though classical rabbinic texts have quite a lot to say about sex and sexuality that is relevant to contemporary sexual questions. Rabbinic discourse is typically wide-ranging, and explicitly sexual subject matter figures into this discourse a fair bit. Furthermore, it appears in frank and sometimes humorous and bawdy terms: the "Fat Rabbis" sugya in Bavli Bava Metsia 84a, for example, compares the penis size of various sages, all of which are ridiculously, comically large. The existence of this frank and ample discussion has no doubt contributed significantly to the prevailing rhetoric of Jewish sex positivity; it has also made it fairly easy and, indeed, intuitive to draw the sorts of one-to-one correspondences between the subject matter of particular texts and contemporary problems that I problematize earlier in this chapter. The matter may perhaps be compared to the phenomenon of attempting to translate mild colloquialisms from one's native language into a new one. The words themselves may literally translate, and the meaning in context may even have something to do with what one is trying to convey, but the overall effect is ultimately quite different.[14]

If, however, these explicitly sexual rabbinic texts are questionable foundations for contemporary claims about values regarding sexual conduct, then what are they doing in the rabbinic canon? Surely the fact that the rabbis considered a frank and wide-ranging discussion of sexuality worthy of inclusion in Oral Torah is significant in some way. Why is it there? What does it accomplish? And what does it tell us about how the rabbis understood sex to function in their textual world?

The last question is the most readily answered, although the answer itself is complex and rather unsatisfying, as the view of sex and sexuality we find in rabbinic sources is, in a word, ambivalent. On the one hand, there are voices that seem quite affirming of sex and sexuality, especially by comparison to many dominant streams within Christianity. On the other hand, there is an equally strong sense in many sources that seems to evince anxiety and caution about sex and sexual desire, particularly as expressed or aroused by women and other marginalized actors.[15] In either case, while we can glean clues about attitudes toward sexuality or about how sexual concerns were or were not woven into Jewish (or proto-Jewish) religious discourse at the time a given text was written or redacted, it is critical to remember that sex is usually not the ultimate subject of discussion.

According to the sexually affirming view, sex is important, even holy, both because it is integral to procreation *and* because it is pleasurable.[16] Thus, for example, a husband has a sexual obligation, or *onah*, to his wife; failure to perform this is considered legitimate grounds for divorce. This obligation is understood as a biblical commandment, based on Exodus 21:10–11: "If he takes himself another wife, he shall not diminish [his first wife's] food, clothing, or sexual rights.[17] If he does not do these three things for her, she shall go freely, without payment." Furthermore, husbands owe their wives a specific schedule of sex, the particulars of which are dependent on his occupation. According to M. Ketubot 5:6, "One who is at leisure [owes his wife sex] daily; laborers, twice weekly; donkey drivers, once weekly; camel drivers, once every thirty days; sailors, once every six months." The next mishnah forbids a husband from taking a vow to abstain from sex with his wife that lasts longer than a week.[18] The Talmudim expand discussion of this issue in different directions. The Yerushalmi takes up the question of occupation, asking whether it is the length of time one spends away from home in one's work or the difficulty of the work that conditions the frequency of a man's obligation to his wife, while the Bavli focuses on the obligations of scholars and the proper balance between devotion to one's wife and devotion to Torah.[19] Interestingly, wives do not have the same sexual obligations toward their husbands; nevertheless, the *moredet*, the "rebellious wife" who refuses sex to her husband, incurs various penalties. M. Ketubot 5:7 states that a moredet suffers a reduction in her ketubah money; the Talmudim understand the moredet specifically as withholding sex, among other things, and expand on the economic penalties she incurs.[20]

According to the sexually cautious view, however, sex, especially sexual temptation as embodied by women, is a source of anxiety and a thing to be eschewed or, at best, very tightly controlled. While, as Satlow puts it, "both men and women were thought to be sexually desirous, [only] men . . . were thought capable of controlling this overwhelming desire."[21] Thus, for example, M. Kidushin 4:12 and 4:14 enjoin men against being secluded with women; these restrictions are also found in the Tosefta and are elaborated in the Talmudim.[22] Stories of sages who are confronted by sexual temptation are common throughout the rabbinic literature. For example, Avot D'Rabbi Natan A16 recounts a series of stories in which sages, while imprisoned by Rome, are sent beautiful women by their captors. In one striking episode, when Rabbi Akiva—who, when sent two beautiful women, is reported to have "[sat] between them, spit, and not turn[ed] to them"—is questioned as to why he did not have sex with the women, he replies, "What could I do? Their odor came over me from the meat of carrion, torn animals, and creeping things." The episode presents Akiva as an exemplar of sagely self-mastery—one who has aligned his will and his desires to the point where what would be irresistibly appealing to most men has become not just morally but sensorially repugnant.

Even in its preferred context—in a marriage to a righteous Jewish woman—sexual expression is, according to this second view, ideally limited and under strict control. Thus, for example, a story in B. Nedarim 20a is what Daniel Boyarin calls a "locus classicus for ascetic sexual practices":[23] "They asked Ima Shalom,[24] the wife of Rabbi Eliezer, 'Why do you have such beautiful children?' She said to them, 'He does not have intercourse with me at the beginning of the night, nor at the end of the night, but at midnight, and when he has intercourse with me, he unveils an inch and veils it again, and appears as if he was driven by a demon.'"[25] Here, to the extent that sex is desirable, it is because of its procreative value. Thus, texts that reflect this second view tend, for example, to connect wives' sexual rights not to sexual pleasure but to the joy surrounding the birth of sons.[26] There is also a significant concern with male self-arousal, one that in later texts becomes explicitly connected to a concern with "wasted seed"—in itself understood as a biblical prohibition. M. Niddah 2:1 states that "every hand that makes frequent examination [of the genitals, for possibly impure discharge]: in a woman, it is praiseworthy, but in a man it should be cut off." The concern here seems to be that checking for discharge will tempt one into masturbation—and note the similarity to the rule about secluding oneself with women, in that one must avoid activities peripheral to the thing that is forbidden so that one's desire does not overcome one. The Bavli on this mishnah goes into a long multipart excursus in which it warns against touching the penis even while urinating, inveighs in strong terms against the wasteful emission of semen, and unequivocally condemns deliberate masturbation. For example, "R. Eliezer said, why is it written, 'your hands are full of blood?' (Isaiah 1:15) These are they who have illicit intercourse with their hands."[27]

Despite the ambivalent views of sex and sexuality found in the rabbinic corpus, however, there are some constants. First, whether a given text tends toward an affirmation of sexuality or an anxiety about it, sexual situations, in almost all cases, are discussed less for their own sake and more as opportunities for the cultivation of discipline, piety, or holiness. Sex in its proper marital context is an opportunity to fulfill *mitsvot*, to establish a well-ordered home and produce children to bring up in piety, and to shape one's desires in a holy direction. Illicit sexual temptation, conversely, is an opportunity to redirect one's mind to Torah, to master base physical urges, and to reaffirm one's commitment to mitsvot. Second, even where sexual variation is acknowledged or even treated leniently, the ideal context for sexual expression remains within a Jewish marriage, and the ideal and defining expression of sexuality is penis-in-vagina (PIV) intercourse, with procreative intent. Again, this is consistent with the first point, that sex functions primarily as a site for the cultivation of specific sagely ideals, ideals that demand the careful regulation of bodily urges such that they can be channeled into particular, acceptable containers. Finally, as with the rabbinic corpus in general, rabbinic discourse on sexuality is conceived and redacted by men, for men, and about men. Women are the focus of this discourse only inasmuch as they present interesting problems for discussion, whether those problems be textual or empirical. Their presence is auxiliary.

Thus, even when we examine explicitly sexual texts in terms of their subject matter, we see that sex in the rabbinic textual world functions less as a multifarious physical appetite that engenders a variety of intimate social interactions that are valuable for their own sake and more as a site of social, familial, and personal formation according to a narrow set of models. Looking at the treatment of sex in rabbinic texts from a hermeneutical perspective, however, further establishes that sex for its own sake is not the rabbis' primary focus. Rather, the ultimate subject of discussion—especially if the source is, as most of them are, linked to the rabbinic tradition—is how to read, interpret, and live out God's Torah. Sexuality, therefore, usually presents itself as a matter for discussion because it is linked in some way to an interpretive problem that the rabbis have raised in their discussion of a given text or because it is a useful site for the formation of the sagely character. Put another way, Jewish sources, even those that *seem* to be about sexuality, are ultimately about *textuality*.

Take, for example, the texts establishing a husband's sexual duty to his wife. As Dorff's work, discussed above, demonstrates, these texts are some of the sources most commonly cited by writers who wish to make a case for Judaism's supposedly fundamental sex positivity. Yet the specifically sexual character of the husband's marital duty becomes a matter for discussion initially because of the ambiguity of the word *onah* in the Exodus text, which, again, stipulates that if a man takes a second wife, he shall not "diminish *she'erah, kesutah*, and *onatah*," usually rendered as "her food, her clothing, and her marital rights." The word *onatah* literally translates to "her time" or "her commerce"—but to what specific time does it refer? Only after this interpretive question comes up for discussion can the verse generate a rabbinic ruling. Indeed, the Mekhilta D'Rabbi Ishmael (a tannaitic midrashic text that is roughly contemporaneous with the mishnah discussed above) on Exodus 21:10 offers three possible interpretations for the meaning of *onatah*:

She'erah—this is her food. And thus it says, "and who eat the *she'er* of my people," (Micah 3:3) and it is written, "He rained *she'er* on them as dust." (Ps. 78:27)

Kesutah—as in its usual sense [i.e., clothing].

And *onatah*—this is her *derekh erets* [lit., "way of the land"; colloq., "the way things are done"; and here, euphemistically, sexual relations], as it is written, "and he lay with her, and *ye'enah*." (Gen. 34:2) These are the words of R. Yoshiah.

R. Yonatan says, *she'erah*—her clothing, clothing that fits her *she'erah* [i.e., her flesh, her body]. If she were young, he should not give her that of an old woman; if she were old, he should not give her that of a girl.

Onatah—he should not give her [clothing] for a warm season during the rainy season, nor should he give her [clothing] for a rainy season during a warm one; rather, he should give her each one in *onatah* [in its time].

From whence "her food?" We learn from a *ḳal v'ḥomer* [roughly, an argument a fortiori]: if he is not permitted to withhold things from her that are not life-sustaining, how much more so is he not permitted to withhold things that are life-sustaining?!

From whence *derekh erets*? We learn from a *ḳal v'ḥomer*: if he is not permitted to withhold from her things for which she was not married to begin with, how much more so does logic indicate that he is not permitted to withhold things for which she *was* married to begin with?!

Rabbi says, *she'erah*—this is *derekh erets*, as it is said, "to all *she'er b'saro*" ["flesh of his flesh," i.e., one is forbidden from sexually approaching one's kin] (Lev 18:6), and it is written, "she is the *she'er* of your father," "she is the *she'er* of your mother" (Lev. 18:12–13).

Kesutah—as in its usual sense.

Onatah—this is her food, as it is stated, "*v'yenacha*, [lit., "and he afflicted you," a different sense of *onah*] and He caused you to hunger." (Deut. 8:3)

Notice that the Mekhilta goes out of its way to highlight the ambiguity of *onah* and *she'er* (which literally means "flesh" but can refer either to the flesh of one's body or to flesh as food), as compared to *kesutah*, which it finds unproblematic. Whenever *kesutah* is mentioned on its own terms, it is tersely glossed as "in its usual sense." Even in Rabbi Yonatan's interpretation, which centers entirely on clothing, *kesutah* is only of interest because of its proximity to the two more ambiguous words. *She'erah* and especially *onatah*, on the other hand, are intriguingly multivalent and so occupy far more of the rabbis' attention. And as a result of this attention, *onah* takes, according to the sages' normative opinion, the meaning of "sexual obligation," not necessarily out of any conviction that women's sexual pleasure is important but because that meaning has acceptable lexical and logical links that harmonize with the sages' interpretations of the other two words. (Indeed, the lexical link through which the sages first establish *onah* as being sexual in character should give pause to any reader assuming sex positivity: Genesis 34 recounts the story of Jacob and Leah's daughter, Dinah, and the most common translation of the *ayin-nun-he* root used there is "rape" or "outrage.")

Another text commonly deployed in the service of a rhetoric of Jewish sex positivity is the episode in Bavli Berakhot 62a in which Rav Kahana (a first-generation Babylonian Amora) hides under the bed of his master, Rav:[28]

> Rav Kahana entered and lay beneath the bed of Rav. He heard him talking and laughing and doing what he required. He said to him, "The mouth of [my teacher] is as one who has never sipped from the dish!" [Rav] said to [Kahana], "Kahana, is that you?! Get out! This is not how we do things!" [It is not *orah ara'a*, the Aramaic analog to *derekh erets*.]
>
> [Kahana] said to him, "It is Torah, and I must learn."

At the outset, one could hardly imagine a more resounding endorsement of the rabbinic valuation of sex. Surely, if a sage compares the study of sexual conduct to the study of Torah, so much so that he feels the need to learn by observing his master in person, sex is of central importance. When one looks more closely, however, this episode starts to sound less like a statement of sex positivity and more like a problem narrative.

To begin with, this narrative occurs within a larger sugya concerned with proper conduct in the privy. Directly preceding the Rav Kahana story are two episodes concerning tannaim and their privy practices:

> It was taught in a *baraita*: Rabbi Akiva said, "I once entered the privy after Rabbi Yehoshua, and I learned three things from it. I learned that one should not face east and west, but rather north and south; I learned that one should not uncover oneself standing, but rather sitting, and I learned that one should not wipe oneself with one's right hand, but rather with one's left."
>
> Ben Azai said to him, "You were insolent with your teacher to this point?!" He said to him, "it is Torah, and I must learn."
>
> It was taught in a *baraita*: Ben Azai said, "I once entered the privy after Rabbi Akiva, and I learned three things from it. I learned that one should not face east and west, but rather north and south; I learned that one should not

uncover oneself standing, but rather sitting, and I learned that one should not wipe oneself with one's right hand, but rather with one's left.

Rabbi Yehuda said to him, "You were insolent with your teacher to this point?!"

He said to him, "it is Torah, and I must learn."

Notice both the similarities and the disjunctions between these two episodes and the Rav Kahana story that directly follows them.[29] All feature a student clandestinely following his master into a private place to learn a lesson, all assume that matters of private, quotidian conduct are important for sagely discipline and learning, and all end with the Hebrew phrase "It is Torah, and I must learn." These establish that the three episodes are clearly part of the same sequence.

Yet there are notable disjunctions, as well. The Aḳiva and Ben Azai narratives are of a piece thematically (the privy), temporally, geographically (they concern tannaim living in Erets Yisrael), and linguistically (Hebrew). They also constitute a transfer of pedagogical tradition among three generations (R. Yehoshua taught R. Aḳiva, who taught Ben Azai), indicating some kind of success for the lesson. Within these stories themselves, furthermore, the student who follows the teacher recounts the story to another; we do not get to see the action itself through the *stam*'s narration. There is also no indication that the student spoke or made his presence known to his teacher in any way.

Compare this to the Rav Kahana story. Here, we see the action as it is occurring from the stam's third-person perspective. The action itself shifts over a century forward and from Erets Yisrael to Babylonia, and the language shifts from Hebrew to Aramaic. The setting shifts from the privy to the bedroom. And there is no transfer of Kahana's practice to the next generation—after this episode, the sugya shifts back to an extended discussion of proper sagely bathroom practices, suggesting that, within the discourse itself, the Kahana story is an unsustainable tangent.

The actual events of the Rav Kahana narrative also differ substantially from the previous two episodes. Aḳiva and Ben Azai are each impressed enough by what they learned from their teachers in the privy to pass the lesson on: each time, the teacher has successfully modeled sagely behavior for the student. But the Rav Kahana episode is marked by mutual disappointment. Kahana is disappointed and shocked that his teacher's sexual conduct is something other than what he expected, although the phrase he uses—"It is as though Aba had never sipped from the dish before!"—is enig-matic. Perhaps he means that Rav appears clumsy and unpracticed in bed or, more likely, that he seems to be too enthusiastic about sex to fit Kahana's idea of sagely decorum. Rav, meanwhile, is (understandably!) appalled that his student has not only invaded his bedroom but does not even have the self-control to keep quiet while doing so. The genre, overall, seems to shift from pedagogical narrative to farce. The previous two narratives emphasized care, control, and minute discipline in even the most private and profane of daily activities. But here, even though Kahana sneaks into Rav's bedroom ostensibly to learn discipline, he cannot maintain it: he blurts out in surprise that his teacher's sexual conduct is far more undisciplined than he had imag-ined, thereby letting loose, as it were, with his own undisciplined ejaculation. The repeated coda that links the three episodes—"It is Torah, and I must learn"—emphasized continuity in the first two episodes, but it becomes an ironic, mocking echo in the third.

If the disjunctions in tone and setting between the three episodes trouble a reading of the Rav Kahana story as an affirmation of rabbinic sex positivity, however, some of the conjunctions between the three episodes trouble that reading even further. For, common to all three episodes is the complete dis-cursive absence of women. We know that the bet midrash was a male space, text study was a male activity, and the formation of the sage was the formation of ideal rabbinic masculinity.[30] In these episodes, we see that even spaces that are *not* the bet midrash are brought under the social norms of that space as they are imported into texts that are concerned with sagely formation. Women, like men, must eliminate; women, like men, participate (indeed, must participate) in partnered sex. The rabbis know this, and elsewhere in the rabbinic corpus they frequently acknowledge it. Here, however, when elimi-nation and sex are considered as potential sites for rabbinic formation, women cease to be relevant.[31] And, in this way, they are treated as similar sorts of phe-nomena. Elimination is done alone; normative rabbinic sex requires a part-ner. Yet even though Rav's wife is there by inference (underscoring yet again the disjunct between the Kahana narrative and the two that precede it), the text seems unwilling to actually flesh her presence out—thereby underscor-ing yet again that this text is less about sex for its own sake (a heterosocial, partnered activity) than it is about sagely study and discipline (a homoso-cial activity). As in the bet midrash, here too—in Rav's bedroom, which unwittingly becomes a failed microcosm of the house of study—women are discursively absent, even when they are physically present.

Moving Forward?

The centrality of text and rabbinic discipline in any rabbinic material means that these textual and formative concerns themselves will substantially determine how that material configures the shape of any empirical phenomenon that may come up for discussion. Thus, anyone wishing to utilize rabbinic text for guidance in matters of contemporary practical ethics—as, indeed, the contemporary discipline of academic Jewish ethics as a whole has decided to do—must look past the simple denominative sense of the words they read in those rabbinic texts to the ways those words are structured. One must seek texts in which either the topics under discussion, or even the formal patterns of the text itself, have substantial relevance to one's questions.

This means that those texts that appear at first to address the very topic on which one seeks guidance may turn out, upon further examination, not to be the best sources of guidance for one's actual questions. Such, I argue, is the case for sex and sexuality. Explicitly sexual texts are not the best analogs for how sex, as a form of social interaction, functions in our contemporary world. Other texts, however, might provide better models.

Text, Form, and Social Function

A serious commitment to Jewish ethics ultimately demands a serious engagement with foundational Jewish texts in one way or another. But, if texts whose subject matter is explicitly sexual are, as I have argued, often poor interlocutors for contemporary questions of sexual ethics, this seems to leave the ethicist who wishes to work with rabbinic texts rather adrift. Subject matter, after all, is a fairly intuitive way to determine whether a given text is relevant to one's project, and, given the vast scope of the classical rabbinic corpus, it is unsustainable to leave the ethicist without any rubric for text selection or textual engagement. But if the surface meaning of a text's subject matter is as a point of interpretive contact both underpowered and overused, how, short of randomly assigning citations to a dartboard, should the hermeneutically sensitive ethicist proceed?

While I am not, in fact, convinced that the dartboard method is wholly without merit (at least as an interpretive exercise), in practice ethicists require ways of selecting texts and methods of engaging with them that possess a stronger internal logic. Fortunately, as I have demonstrated, there is always far more going on in these texts than indicated by their simple subject matter alone, and it is in this material that lies just below the surface that one can recover a number of alternative hermeneutics, several of which may promise more nuanced, generative, and potentially liberatory possibilities for contemporary moral discourse than what the simple denominative sense of the subject matter can provide.

In what follows, I discuss some of the basic parameters of what I consider sustainable and hermeneutically sensitive methods of contemporary ethical engagement with rabbinic text. I then explicate in somewhat more detail two specific approaches to such engagement that I consider especially promising. The second of these approaches—drawing comparisons between the respective social functions of the rabbinic subject matter and the contemporary problem—I explicate further and then employ, using two case studies, in part II of the book.

Features of Empirically Sensitive Methods of Engagement

I propose that a method of textual engagement that cultivates the virtues of empirical justice and hermeneutic competency—by which I mean a mode of engaging classical texts with contemporary moral questions in a way that is aware of and responsive to the empirical details of both the text and the contemporary phenomenon—should have the following characteristics. First, it should try to stay true to the text as such without either revising or apologizing for its more problematic content. Second, it should demand an attentiveness to context, form, and style that is good practice for any reader. Third, it should help articulate a way of doing ethics that is particularly and substantially in conversation with the tradition from which it arises, while nevertheless being able to helpfully contribute to ethical discourses outside of that tradition.

By "staying true to the text as such," I mean that an empirically just mode of engagement should understand and acknowledge that the world we find in classical texts is by and large one that is socially, philosophically, and morally alien. This is not to say that there are *no* significant conceptual continuities between rabbinic texts and modern systems of thought, politics, and law; a number of scholars, for example, have pointed out numerous ways in which Talmudic legal reasoning has influenced modern American legal reasoning.[32]

It is, however, to say that the rabbis operated under concepts of class, subjectivity, gender, and sexuality that are often incongruous with or even contradictory of commitments that readers with liberationist aims hold contemporarily, and readers should not pretend otherwise. This does not mean that readers must jettison their normative aims—doing so, after all, would render the entire discipline of practical ethics moot. Nor does it mean that readers may not engage in consciously acknowledged and flagged acts of deliberately anachronistic counterreading to elucidate or expand a potential avenue of inquiry.[33] It does mean, however, that scholars must be careful to avoid claiming the rabbis as, say, "sex positive," "protofeminist," or "death penalty abolitionists." They were none of these things; these are modern concepts that would have made no sense to them or to their contemporaries. They may well have had certain concerns about women's well-being that seem to us progressive by comparison to some of their contemporaries, or they may not have, but this is not evidence of their somehow having anticipated a fundamentally modern agenda.

An empirically just reader, then, must accept that they have chosen to deal with texts that will often clash with or be incomprehensible to their own values. They may choose to deal with that clash in any number of ways, and in the following section, I discuss ways of engaging with the troubling features of classical texts in more detail. For now, it is enough to note that the empirically just ethicist must neither excuse nor elide them.

By "attentiveness to context, form, and style," I mean that, even beyond acknowledging the fundamental particularity of the moral and social content of the text in front of them, the empirically sensitive ethicist must also attend to the mechanics through which that content is addressed and what content surrounds the content on which one focuses. It is not enough, in other words, to simply note *that* a text has troubling (or appealing!) content; one must also give some attention to the way in which that content is reached, explicated, and presented within the textual world, as well as to its sociohistorical background and context, where available. As I discussed in the previous section, considering a text that, in isolation, seems to be evidence of rabbinic sex positivity, in light of its narrative context, the textual problems that generate it, and the way in which it is reasoned and redacted, casts the meaning of that text in a whole new light.

By "articulating a mode of doing ethics that is particularly and substantially in conversation with the tradition from which it arises," I mean that the empirically just reader should draw on methods of reading and interpreting their canon that are grounded in some form of traditional practice, although they need not by any means copy them wholesale. This follows to a great extent from the previous virtue, for both share the belief that *how* a text is formed, explicated, presented, and discussed is equally significant (if not, in many cases, more so!) as the subject matter of that text; here, I state explicitly that a great part of what makes a text sacred and locates it in a tradition is how its readers interact with it. Judaism and Christianity, for example, share the canon of texts variously called the Hebrew Bible, the Tanakh, or the Old Testament; what distinguishes a Tanakh from an Old Testament, even though they might contain exactly the same words, is how readers have interacted with them and how they continue to do so. These layers of interpretive history and reading practice subsequently accrete to the text and become a part of that text's life. So if one wants to play with that set of words *as the Tanakh*, one must accept that one is actually playing with more than those words. One is playing with centuries upon centuries of rich and generative interpretive history that cannot be discarded; what's more, that history has particular and helpful lessons for the contemporary ethicist.

Yet even though I call for the ethicist who locates themselves in a particular tradition to be grounded in and in conversation with that tradition's textual practices, it does not follow that I believe the ethicist located within a particular tradition must be limited or parochial in scope. The moral problems we face in the present day are rarely limited in consequence to a particular interpretive community, and the insights traditional texts and methods of reading may offer are not necessarily limited in application to that community, either. The challenge is to speak beyond one's particularity while nevertheless remaining flexibly rooted within it.

One Method: Attending to the Moral Significance of a Text's Formal Structure

One possibility, articulated by Emily Filler, is to use rabbinic—and biblical—texts in a formalist way: rather than drawing ethical conclusions about their content, one uses the ways rabbinic texts work through issues as models for ways of thinking about contemporary issues. Filler contests the assumption that there is a way of deploying classical texts to do ethical work that is fundamentally stable across religious traditions.[34] Rather, she argues, the very structure of classical Jewish texts nudges the reader not only into interpreting those texts differently than one would interpret texts from other traditions but also into a different mode of ethical reasoning. For her, "as much as any-thing, it is the *way* this content appears which defines [classical texts]—and defines the way they work (or do not work) in Jewish ethics."[35] Features of classical texts, such as the Gemara's preservation of pitched and polyvocal debate or narrative midrash's recognition of multiple possible meanings or interpretations of a biblical word or phrase, not only militate against univo-cal methods of interpretation; they trouble the assumption that the Jewish ethicist should seek singular, discrete, text-based solutions to contemporary ethical problems to begin with.[36]

Filler's approach has the three virtues I have listed above. Additionally, it encourages the writer to think outside of the often narrow canon of texts heretofore employed by academic Jewish ethicists on their topic of choice. If the form rather than the content is primary, any subject matter may be arranged in such a way that it is a potential source of guidance for a given problem. This method is a valuable tool for the contemporary Jewish ethicist, and further, I think that Filler is likely correct when she claims that a primary focus on the form rather than the content of classic texts "can aid Jewish ethicists in employing these texts in ways . . . which are more distinctively *Jewish*."[37] By this, I think Filler means that (a) the classical texts that are sub-stantially formative of rabbinic Judaism and upon which Jewish ethicists rely a great deal are often ultimately *about* formal matters of law or hermeneutics more so than they are about their apparent subject matter, and (b) there is something characteristically Jewish about the particular modes of interpret-ation and discourse found in rabbinic text. When contemporary ethicists attend to the texts' emphasis on form and participate in the particular modes of discourse demonstrated by those texts, they are performing "distinctively Jewish" ways of doing ethics.

Another Method: Attending to the Social Function of the Text's Subject Matter

That said, I do not believe that a strictly formalist approach is the *only* her-meneutical method that possesses the virtues I have enumerated available to the practical ethicist. Just because one cannot assume a one-to-one corres-pondence between the content of a rabbinic text and a contemporary ethical problem does not mean that the content is *completely* alien to contemporary concerns or that it cannot do any useful work for a particular problem. When Berkowitz examines rabbinic descriptions of the ritual of capital punishment, she asks, in a Foucauldian mode, "What work does this ritual of execution do? How is capital punishment mobilized? What is the political significance of [the rabbinic] reluctance to execute and concern to preserve the body?"[38] Berkowitz is asking, in other words, about the *social function* of execution rituals in the world of rabbinic discourse. How do these rituals generate and maintain rabbinic power? What do they reveal about the limits of that power? More broadly, what do the particulars of these rituals—the specific forms of execution they mandate, the ways they manage space and time, silence and speech—tell us about the workings of a world of complex and multilayered interactions between person and person, person and state, person and expert authority as the rabbis understood it?

Berkowitz asks these questions in the capacity of a text scholar and historian, but I contend that this type of inquiry into the functional details of cases within rabbinic text—an approach I shall refer to as "functionalist"—can be equally useful for the practical ethicist.[39] If we want to work with rabbinic content, and we accept the claim that the ultimate subject matter of rabbinic text is the rabbis and their world, the next question should be, "How do the specific phenomena the rabbis discuss function within the world of rabbinic text?" Along these lines, when one employs rabbinic text to address a contemporary problem, the way that problem functions in its contemporary context may serve as a guiding rubric by which to examine rabbinic texts. Texts that may initially appear unrelated to the contemporary problem may prove, upon more careful examination of the work their subject matter does, to address questions that are highly germane, because their subject matter may function similarly to that of the problem at hand. Thus, sex in rabbinic text has, as a rule, different social functions than does sex in the contemporary world—but there may be *other* matters discussed in other rabbinic texts that function similarly to aspects of contemporary sexuality.

Such a functionalist approach makes it relatively difficult to make generalizing claims about "what or how the rabbis thought," because it is necessarily case based and because its primary objects of inquiry are the details of particular phenomena in their textual context.[40] It is not concerned with making sweeping moral claims on behalf of the rabbis; rather, it does its moral work by first identifying the ways the rabbis construe certain phenomena as functioning socially, ritually, and morally and then carefully comparing those construals of function to social, ritual, and moral aspects of the contemporary problem under discussion. If the subject matter of the rabbinic text, or "source," and that of the contemporary ethical problem, or "target," turn out to reproduce similar structures of social interaction or authority, or if they illuminate similar aspects of types of interaction people engage in or of the world they inhabit, then that particular source is likely to be a fruitful basis for constructive work on that particular target.[41]

This comparison of the social, ritual, and moral functions of the rabbinic source and the contemporary target, in turn, provides a basis for the ethicist to ask how the contemporary situation might improve practically and morally. Such a comparison might suggest that particulars of the rabbinic analogue's function may be an improvement on the ways we currently conceive of and address contemporary problem. It may also be the case that problems in the functioning of the rabbinic analog may serve to elucidate comparable problems in the contemporary situation. In addition, this approach acknowledges Filler's caution against using a single set of interpretive techniques across different canons for which they may not be equally suited. It also shares her concern with *how* content is deployed rather than simply asking *what* the content is.

"The rabbis," writes Berkowitz, "are not a simple resource for either side of the contemporary death penalty debate. They *are* a resource, however, for better understanding the workings of authority, its strategies of persuasion, and the role that violence plays in those strategies."[42] Contemporary sexual ethics, and the texts we use to think about them, largely raise different functional questions than does rabbinic discourse on the rituals of execution (although, as we shall see in chapter 5, rabbinic discourse on execution does raise questions about the relationship between performativity and power that are quite germane to sexual ethics), but Berkowitz's broader caution about how to employ rabbinic discourse as a contemporary reader rings as true here as it does there. The rabbis are not simple resources for any side in contemporary debates about sexual ethics, Jewish or otherwise. But they may be invaluable, if complex resources for understanding the workings of social interaction and social risk—an understanding that, in turn, may help us develop better ways to manage risks while continuing to act as the fundamentally social beings that we are.

Toward an Ethics of Textual Relation

This is a chapter about hermeneutics and rabbinic text, one that forms the center of a book about sexual ethics and about the ethics of relationship more broadly. The book has discussed and continues to discuss the ethics of relationship; in this chapter, it has discussed the ethics of interpretation. But these, as I hope is now becoming clear, are not mutually exclusive subjects. Rather, each category (relationship and interpretation) applies to and is intertwined with each subject (sex and rabbinic text) because there are better and worse ways of relating to a sexual partner, and there are better and worse ways of interpreting a text. But there are also better and worse ways of interpreting the phenomenon of sex, and there are better and worse ways of relating to text as a dialogue partner.

For the relationship between the sacred text and the interpreter is, precisely, a dialogical relationship in which each member affects and makes moral demands on the other. As Steven Kepnes argues regarding Martin Buber's hermeneutics, "the Bible"—and I see no reason this does not extend to other sacred texts as well—"can be regarded as a Thou and the process of interpretation phrased as a 'dialogue' with the text. . . . With the *Mikra* [the written Torah], we understand how one can have a 'conversation' with a text as one has with a person."[43] This relationship is not flattening or totalizing. The text and its interpreters remain distinct entities who can and do clash: "The horizon of the text and that of the reader are never 'fused,' as Gadamer would wish, but are held in vibrating tension like the bold patches of color that jut up against one another in the paintings of Mark Rothko."[44] Nor is this conversation a closed circuit; rather, "the interpretation of a text is a matter of dialogue not only between the reader and the text but also between the reader and fellow interpreters."[45] And, because the text *is* a Thou who demands respect, it follows both that it is possible to do interpretive violence to the text and that the text makes the moral demand of its reader *not* to do such violence, to "respect this book as a product of a dialogue of a human being and a form of spirit. . . . The face of the author . . . hovers over the text and prohibits the interpreter from severing the text from the concrete life of dialogue and the human suffering and joy out of which the text arose."[46]

The whole of this book, then, is ultimately about relational ethics. Sex is an intimate and risk-laden mode of relating to other human beings, and hermeneutics is an intimate and risk-laden mode of relating to texts. In each case, there are better and worse ways of engaging in that relation—ways that are mutual and well negotiated and ways that are unilateral and coercive, ways that foster growth and ways that foster stagnation. In what follows, I suggest ways of relating to the phenomenon of sex that I judge to foster good hermeneutical practice; or, conversely, I suggest hermeneutical practices that I judge to be more likely to foster good ways of relating to the phenomenon of sex and, I hope, good sexual practice in and of itself.

Ancient Texts' and Contemporary Concerns' Relationship Status: It's Complicated

One core relational question that has animated this chapter concerns the relationship between present-day ethical-normative concerns and rabbinic texts. I have been critical of what I perceive as one dominant mode of relation between these present-day concerns and rabbinic texts. This posture, however, ought not be misunderstood as indicating that I believe that such concerns must never color our interpretations of classical texts. On the contrary, I believe such complete objectivity is impossible. No matter how carefully we attempt to occupy a position of studied and serious academic detachment, we will always be particular people, with particular formative experiences and core commitments, when we encounter those texts, and there is no way for those commitments and experiences, at some level, not to color our encounter with the texts and to inform our understanding of what kind of entities those texts are. The influence of contemporary concerns on our understanding of rabbinic reasoning, furthermore, is not unidirectional. Just as our contemporary commitments and the practical issues we face as contemporary reasoners affect the ways we read rabbinic texts, so, too, do the reasoning patterns we excavate as a result of our interactions with rabbinic texts affect the ways we "read" our contemporary issues. Rabbinic texts come out of a different time and place, but we read them with eyes all our own, so they become different entities than they were in their original contexts. And when we condition our minds through the practice of reading those texts, the contemporary problems we consider take different shapes when viewed through the lens of that mental conditioning. As Kepnes argues, "as in any form of I-Thou relationship, one cannot leave a true encounter with the biblical text"—or any sacred text—"without being existentially affected."[47]

This is not to say that there is, therefore, no way in which we, as scholars, can discipline our encounters with these texts so that the texts may have some chance to speak "for themselves." On the contrary, the fact that we have particular experiences and commitments that unavoidably shape our encounters with and interpretations of texts is an important datum in our processes of textual analysis. By paying attention to the particular ways in which our experiences unavoidably shape our interaction with the text, and how that interaction in turn shapes our perspective going forward, we can discipline our interpretive practices that much more carefully. We cannot excise the influence of our standpoint on our interpretation, but we can understand it and channel it.

This matter also affects how to answer the question of whether rabbinic reasonings have useful things to say to contemporary moral problems. I argue that they do but that how well they address them depends on how we, as contemporary readers, discipline our interpretations. If we are cognizant of the ways our standpoints affect our readings and, conversely, of the standpoints offered by the texts themselves, then those texts can offer valuable if sometimes unexpected resources for addressing contemporary problems.

On Morally Troubling Texts

Thinking about our reading practices in terms of dynamic interpersonal relationships also has critical implications for how we deal with morally and politically troubling texts. While the rabbis' understanding of sex and sexuality is so morally and socially dissonant with our current understanding as to have become, as I have argued, practically a different phenomenon, we as contemporary readers will not avoid moral and political dissonance with our texts merely by seeking out closer functional parallels to our questions. Indeed, using different texts, more likely than not, raises different and potentially more complicated moral concerns about their history, form, and content. However, in raising these new concerns or raising older concerns in new ways, rabbinic texts, in dialogue with contemporary questions, may help us think through moral problems in ways we did not anticipate when we began the dialogue.

It is hardly a novel observation that rabbinic literature, especially in light of contemporary moral sensibilities, is insular, elitist, and androcentric. As I noted above, rabbinic literature, before it is about anything else, is about

rabbis and the place of rabbis in the world as they saw it. And since the rabbis were at once Jews living as an underclass in a world often hostile to them,
elites within the Jewish community (or at least, the rabbis understood themselves as an elite class) who were trying to establish their understanding of
Judaism as normative, and men living in a patriarchal world, it follows that
rabbinic literature overwhelmingly reflects those biases. To use this literature fully and responsibly, one must on some level engage its failings as well as
its strengths. Further, the rabbis' insularity, elitism, and sexism are not so far
removed from contemporary discourse as we would perhaps like to believe.
Thus, examining specific ways these failings function in rabbinic text may
provide insight into how similar moral failings function today.

Take, for example, ritual purity texts, which I use in chapter 4, to think
about STIs. These texts have several features that are surprisingly consonant
with a contemporary and even liberatory understanding of sex, sociality, and
public health: they model matter-of-fact dialogue about potentially embar-
rassing bodily issues, they treat contagion as an unavoidable consequence of
social intercourse that is everyone's concern, and they offer a management
strategy based on self-examination and self-awareness. At the same time,
however, these texts deploy specific troubling discourses about Gentiles,
amei ha'arets ("people of the land," a group whose identity is the subject of
some debate but who at the very least can be understood as nonrabbinic Jews
whom the rabbis disdained), and women.

Gentiles do not become personally impure as a consequence of touching
an impure object or experiencing a condition, such as scale disease or genital discharge, that would render a Jew impure. At the same time, however,
Gentiles convey impurity to people and objects and are not allowed contact
with holy things. As Mira Balberg puts it, "Whereas a Jew is 'pure' in the sense
that she attains or maintains a state of purity, a Gentile is [unable to contract
impurity] because she is outside the realm of impurity altogether."[48] Simultaneously, however, Gentiles "are considered to be *inherently* impure due to
the very fact that they are not Jews, and this inherent impurity cannot be
gotten rid of until the Gentile actively converts to Judaism. . . . In the rabbinic
system Gentiles are both categorically pure and categorically impure."[49]

That Gentiles are categorically *pure* illustrates that the ability to contract
impurity is actually a sign of high status within the rabbinic system. Because
the rabbinic purity system functions as a school for the cultivation of a self

that is disciplined and attentive to the rules of purity and to the bodily states, social interactions, and physical and temporal conditions that affect one's purity status, a person who is susceptible to impurity is one who has a sense of self that is susceptible to discipline. As Balberg puts it, "The notion that Gentiles are not susceptible to impurity serves . . . to tell Jews something about what they are and what they ought to be: that which turns them into agents, that which allows them to act as willful and conscious subjects and thus partake in the shaping of their world, is their subordination to the Torah."[50]

Yet if the Gentile's insusceptibility to impurity is a sign that they lack a self that is susceptible to discipline, their simultaneous constant ritual impurity—that is, they are able to transmit impurity to others—demonstrates the results of not disciplining the self. The Gentile, unlike the ideal rabbinic subject, is understood to be uncontrolled and undisciplined—something that is underscored perhaps most strongly by the explicit comparison of the ritual impurity of Gentiles to that of a *zav* (a man with an irregular penile discharge, about whom more in chapter 4) in Tosefta Zavim 2:1: "The Gentiles, the convert, and the resident alien are not susceptible to *zivah* impurity, but even though they are not susceptible to *zivah* impurity, they are impure, like a *zav*, in every respect. They burn *terumah* on their account, but they are not liable for rendering impure the sanctuary or its holy things."[51] Balberg reads the comparison between the Gentile and the zav to have important rhetorical implications regarding rabbinic subjectivity, regardless of how completely the tannaitic system cashes out the analogy.[52] Since, as she argues, the tannaitic purity system is a site for the rabbinic subject to practice self-examination and especially self-*control*, it is noteworthy that Gentiles are compared to a man who experiences an *uncontrollable* genital flux. A man with uncontrollable, continuous discharge "is thus a man whose form of impurity is comparable to that of a woman."[53] The tannaim, Balberg argues, carry this even further: for them, at least according to some sources, "the *zav* . . . is in certain ways a man *who has turned into a woman*. The Rabbis assert that men with abnormal genital discharges . . . must constantly scrutinize and examine their genitalia in the same way that women do."[54] Thus, by comparing Gentiles to *zavim*, Balberg argues, the tannaim are essentially "associat[ing] non-Jews with deficient masculinity."[55]

Gentiles are not the only class associated with a lack of self-control in tannaitic purity discourse. The amei ha'arets are primarily identified within the

Mishnah by "their notable carelessness regarding impurity, at least according to rabbinic standards."[56] The amei ha'arets are assumed to be perpetually impure, not because they exist outside the rabbinic system and thus *cannot* become pure (like Gentiles) but because of "their insufficient efforts to maintain a state of purity in their everyday lives."[57] Mishnah Ṭaharot 7:3, for example, assumes that when workers from among the amei ha'arets have been left unattended inside one's home, some significant portion of its contents will be rendered impure. This and other passages not only assume ritual impurity on the part of the amei ha'arets but also assume, per Balberg, that they cannot resist touching things; M. Ṭaharot 7:4 describes women from this group as compulsively "touching" or "meddling" with items in a pure house.[58] Such inattention to the rules of purity and inability to resist touching things is also a characteristic of children: that the amei ha'arets "meddle" with things "resonates with a mishnaic ruling that since it is a child's way to touch whatever it sees, whenever a child is found next to dough, the dough should be considered impure.[59] Like children, then, the People of the Land conduct themselves in respect to impurity in a way that can be best described as *mindlessness*."[60] So if Gentiles lack the susceptibility to discipline that comes from willed subjection to the Torah, the amei ha'arets lack a different sort of susceptibility to discipline, a lack that seems to come from some more basic deficiency in executive function. They are compared to children, where Gentiles are compared to women, or at least to womanlike men. In either case, each group is construed as other and compared unfavorably to the self-aware, self-controlled rabbinic subject.

Of course, the fact that femininity is a point of unfavorable comparison and that it is contrasted unfavorably with the rabbinic ideal of self-control also bears examination. As I have noted, rabbinic discourse was created by, for, and about rabbis, which is to say it was created by, for, and about men. The mishnaic subject who strives toward purity is a male subject. This is clear, Balberg argues, not only because the Mishnah was created "for men by men" but because "the purity of women in the Mishnah is always presented as instrumental to the purity of men. . . . Moreover, the Rabbis of the Mishnah define women's commitment to purity strictly in terms of the commitment of their male guardians, either their husbands or their fathers. . . ."[61] Even though women can potentially strive to develop the qualities of the mishnaic idealized subject, this ideal subject is clearly a male."[62] The default subject is male, and this default, idealized subject is characterized by a commitment to purity that manifests itself in physical and psychological self-control. Such qualities are thereby cast as *masculine* qualities, an association that is made explicit when we compare texts that deal with women's purity practices. Women are assumed to have inferior self-control, both physiologically (like a zav, since menstruation, their paradigmatic impurity, is an uncontrolled genital flux) and psychologically (like the amei ha'arets, who are assumed to be unable to resist touching things they ought not touch). Balberg cites a case in M. Ṭaharot 7:9 in which R. Akiva declares that if a woman is cooking *terumah* in a pot, leaves the pot unattended, and upon her return finds another woman feeding coals to the first woman's fire, the terumah is presumed impure because "women are greedy, and she is suspected of uncovering her friend's pot to know what she is cooking." As the amei ha'arets are assumed to be unable to refrain from touching what they ought not touch, so too are women assumed to be unable to keep from assuaging their curiosity. Both groups are infantilized since, as noted above, the inability to touch what one ought not touch is considered the characteristic of a child.

Similarly, even in a purity system that assumes the default state of the body to be porous and modular, the leakiness of women's bodies is singular because it is a leakiness that defies easy interpretability. Typical female leakage is uncontrolled, whereas typical male leakage is controlled: the paradigm case for male genital impurity is seminal emission (*ḳeri*)—a single, momentary, theoretically controllable emission—while the paradigm case of female genital impurity is menstruation (*niddah*), a continuous, protracted, uncontrollable flux. As Balberg puts it, "The seeping and unruly nature of women's bodies makes them more prone to impurity not only because such bodies are harder to control, but also because such bodies are more difficult to *know*."[63] That these bodies are more difficult to know is a result not only of the uncontrollability of their seepage but also of its location. Rabbinic discourse characterizes female genital impurity as *bivśarah*, "in her flesh," and male genital impurity as *mivśaro*, "from his flesh."[64] Typical male leakage and impurity is characterized as external and therefore more immediately knowable or interpretable. Typical female leakage and impurity, however, is characterized as internal. It is therefore in need of professional interpretation. And since knowledge, for the rabbis, is intimately linked to authority, women's bodies become simultaneously less governable for the women who inhabit them and more in need of governing by sagely authorities.

This governance finds its most complex and developed expression in the rules surrounding menstrual impurity (niddah). Charlotte Fonrobert, in her pivotal work *Menstrual Purity: Rabbinic and Christian Reconstructions of Biblical Gender*, argues that the complex taxonomy of bloodstains enumerated in Mishnah Niddah constitutes a "rabbinic 'science' of women's blood," which functions as a kind of scaffold for rabbinic authority structures.[65] Not all genital discharges in men are true *zivah*; similarly, not all female genital bleeding is true niddah. M. Niddah 2:6–7 sets forth a schema of colors that have various implications for purity status.[66] Within the realm of female genital bleeding, there is the impurity of the niddah (regular menstruation) and that of the *zavah* (irregular genital bleeding), and in each subtype, a number of variations in blood color can lead to a diagnosis of impurity. Where female bleeding is concerned, Fonrobert argues that this complexity—which makes the blood a subject of academic debate among male scholars—"entirely [displaces women] from the scene."[67] The disembodied blood itself is the topic of conversation.

Fonrobert takes particular notice of the fact that the determination of impurity is made visually. In a rabbinic innovation that differs from biblical law, blood variations are examined and impurity determined by way of stains (*ketem*) on cloth, whether the examiner is the woman herself (in the case of normal menstruation) or a rabbi (in the case of a doubt as to the status of the bleeding). The leakiness and unpredictability of women's bodies—and, more critically here, the internal location of the relevant leaks—make those bodies less knowable. Given the inscrutability of the bodies—the sources of the blood—the rabbis focus on visual inspection of stains on an external object, Fonrobert argues, because they "had no direct access to the woman's body itself [and] could establish control based on external evidence more readily and more 'objectively' than on the blood flow itself. . . . The inspection of a bloodstain or blood on a testing rag to be judged by a rabbinic expert is another way for rabbinic discourse to objectify menstrual bleeding."[68]

Furthermore, the characterization of female leakage as internal gives rise to an extended rabbinic metaphor in which the female body, especially the reproductive body, is characterized as a house. M. Niddah 2:5, for example, explicitly analogizes the female reproductive system as consisting of a "vestibule, a chamber, and an upper chamber." In addition to establishing that the female body is a body that is meant to be occupied—if the nature of the female body is interior, that body is meant to be dwelt in, and the appropriate occupant is the woman's husband—this metaphor also establishes that the female body is an inanimate object and thereby subject to *objective* analysis. As Elizabeth Shanks Alexander has put it, "if the woman's body is an inanimate object, she is not uniquely positioned to determine what is happening within it."[69]

Rabbinic legal expertise concerning the onset of menstruation and the purity of a given bloodstain thus supersedes the sensations and experience of the actual person who is bleeding; indeed, legal categories themselves sometimes seem to supersede physical evidence. Fonrobert and Chaya Halberstam both examine a case in M. Niddah 3:8 in which a woman, suspecting irregular bleeding, brings a dubious bloodstain before Rabbi Akiva:

> It happened that a woman came before Rabbi Akiva, and said to him, "I saw a bloodstain."
> He said to her, "Perhaps you had an internal wound?"
> She said to him, "Yes, but it healed."
> He said to her, "Perhaps it could have been reopened, and let out blood?"
> She said to him, "Yes . . ."
> Rabbi Akiva declared her pure.
> He saw his students looking at one another, and said to them, "Why is this matter difficult in your eyes? The sages did not say this to be stringent, but rather to be lenient, as it says: 'When a woman has a discharge, her discharge being blood in her flesh' (Lev. 15:19)—*blood*, and not *stain!*"

In explicating the Levitical verse as he does, Akiva privileges a specific process of interpreting both the biblical text and the "text" of the bloodstain over the woman's observations regarding her physical history. In fact, Halberstam argues, he goes even further: he "effects a radical separation between blood and bloodstain, defusing the evidentiary force of the bloodstain by declaring it utterly meaningless within biblical law, and viable in rabbinic law only in cases of virtual certainty."[70] In other words, the biblical law demands actual blood, and since Akiva is operating within rabbinic law—which privileges the stain over actual blood—cases with even a modicum of doubt are judged leniently. Akiva "privileges a mere possibility (perhaps the wound reopened?) over a known fact (it healed)."[71]

Fonrobert reads this as a clear case of the rabbinic system of expertise in blood establishing authority over and against the physical experience of the one who bleeds.[72] Halberstam agrees that this case represents an assertion of rabbinic authority but in a subtler fashion. Rather than simply separating the blood from the woman and treating it as disembodied evidence, Halberstam argues, Akiva entirely abstracts the *legal* category of ketem from the physical reality of a bloodstain on a piece of cloth: "R. Aqiba does not determine that she has an internal wound; he merely inquires into the possibility, and makes a *legal* decision that she is ritually pure."[73] Thus, a layperson's—and, significantly, a lay*woman's*—observation of an empirical reality bears only distant relation to the rules she must follow in the social reality created by the rabbis. Knowability is authority; the focus on the doubtfulness of basic empirical knowledge creates a space for its supersession by abstract legal knowledge, which, in turn, establishes spaces of power for the class that has privileged access to that legal knowledge.

Thus, by examining the ways these three groups—gentiles, amei ha'arets, and especially women—are rendered as other in the purity texts, it becomes clear, especially from the perspective of purity's use in practical ethics, that the undergirding concern here is the pervasive question of authority. The tannaitic rabbis treat impurity as a day-to-day issue whose management involves a process of self-discipline and self-formation, but they do so in a way that maintains a central, indispensable role for rabbinic authority, an authority that is inescapably gendered.[74] This is primarily because the ideal rabbinic subject is already male. Furthermore, menstrual impurity is a major part of purity discourse—indeed, it is the only form of ritual impurity that retains practical import in modern Judaism—and provides particularly fertile ground for the exercise of rabbinic authority, as Balberg, Halberstam, and especially Fonrobert have shown.

The rabbis' treatment of outsiders, then—and their consolidation of authority such that it rests only with the originators of their own specific form of legal discourse—is not something to emulate in and of itself. Reading and discussing this treatment, however, *can* illuminate ways in which in-group/out-group dynamics, the hoarding of authoritative discourse, and the ways in which minoritized groups are treated by legal and medical authorities function in our present contexts. Furthermore, as I discuss more extensively in chapter 5, rabbinic discourses of authority, read in light of their liminal position of power, can shed particular light on the ways groups that are privileged in some respects and marginalized in others variously reproduce, appropriate, modify, and in some respects consciously queer oppressive structures of authority.

Disciplines of Reading and Relation

How, then, to discipline our reading? And what might these unexpected textual resources look like? To begin with, I would argue that the first discipline that flows from the reading practices I have suggested throughout this chapter is the simple recognition that not only my values but even—and, I would suggest, more importantly—my ontological understandings of the phenomena under discussion are at least in part alien to the texts' understandings of those phenomena. This may seem a truism, but the beginning of an honest and ethical conversation of any kind is the acknowledgment that it is necessarily occurring across some kind of difference. Such acknowledgment thus recognizes the ever-present possibility of misunderstanding and error and so (one hopes) acts as at least a partial check against interpretive hubris.

By the same token, by consenting to work with these texts in spite of the above-acknowledged differences, I am also acknowledging the possibility that a perspective that is at least partly alien to my own, morally and ontologically, may nevertheless have something of value to teach me regarding the problem I am attempting to address. That is, by consenting to engage, I am also consenting to the possibility of being taught and thereby being changed, corrected, and unsettled by this alien perspective.

Because I have acknowledged that the texts' ontological understanding may be alien to mine, I can thus be open to the possibility that the resources that may be most helpful for my current problem are not necessarily where I would first expect them to be. It is not just that the rabbis' values about sexuality are different from mine; it is that the rabbis understood sexuality to be a different sort of thing than I understand it to be. By the same token, however, the rabbis understood social contagion to be a different sort of thing than I am used to understanding it as—and because I have acknowledged that the texts' perspective is alien to mine in some important ways, I can also be open to the possibility that the text permits connections between phenomena that the perspective with which I encountered the text might have precluded.

Another critical discipline here is to have a thorough understanding of where one's own moral and ontological convictions are more and less likely to give. I know myself, as a human and as a scholar, well enough to know that my own basic beliefs about the nature of sex and, by extension, about sexual morality are unlikely to conform to those I find in rabbinic text, not least because those views are formed by my own lived experience as a queer woman. By knowing what my convictions are and where they came from, I am better able to sort out my own convictions from those I see in the text and to evaluate the latter on something slightly closer to their own terms. I also know, however, that I am far less committed to a particular moral and ontological understanding of other aspects of social intercourse, and so I am therefore more open to being shaped and taught by the texts regarding those aspects.

None of these practices are, by themselves, sufficient for doing good text work or good constructive ethics; nor will they result in work that manages to remain perfectly faithful to the texts' original intent (whatever that may be) while still neatly solving contemporary problems. They are, however, helpful and important practices for religious ethicists who wish to use rabbinic texts in this way. They also establish that the practice of using religious texts to address contemporary problems is not a unidirectional relationship but rather a conversation. Rabbinic texts are not resources to be mined; they are dialogue partners, with perspectives, needs, and difficulties of their own, and many of the moral rules that apply to interacting with flesh-and-blood others also apply to interacting with them. The encounter with rabbinic text is one from which no party comes away unaltered.

2. SOCIAL INTERCOURSE

Why Sex Is Enmeshed in Sociality

IF HALF OF MY argument in this book is that we cultivate specific, broadly applicable virtues when we read sex in contiguity with other social interactions, empirical justice and hermeneutic competency demand that I carefully examine those contiguities. In this chapter, I lay out the ways sexual interaction exists in descriptive and normative entanglement with other forms of social relation and show why many of the putative moral boundaries between sex and other forms of sociality are not just artificial but actually harmful.

For scholars of gender and sexuality, the claim that sex is a species of social relation is hardly a novel one.[1] As Gayle Rubin has put it, "Sexuality is as much a human product as are diets, methods of transportation, systems of etiquette, forms of labor, types of entertainment, processes of production, and modes of oppression."[2] And, more broadly, Audre Lorde's classic essay "Uses of the Erotic" argues that the channeling of the erotic, which is "a measure between the beginnings of our sense of self and the chaos of our strongest feelings . . . an internal sense of satisfaction to which, once we have experienced it, we know we can aspire,"[3] into a very narrow definition of sex functions to cordon off other aspects of life into discrete boxes, effectively separating political power from any affective parts of human experiences. "All sexuality," as anthropologist Margot Weiss argues, "is a social relation, linking subjects (individuals, desires, and embodiments) to socieconomics (social hierarchies, communities, and relations of inequality)."[4] Sexuality, as the Christian womanist ethicist Kelly Brown Douglas argues, drawing on the Christian ethicist James Nelson, also "compels our emotional, affective, sensual, and spiritual relationships."[5] Sexual interactions are integral parts of broader structures of power and social order, and the norms cultivated in sexual interactions affect and are affected by these broader structures.

Scholars of religious ethics, however—with notable exceptions like Kelly Brown Douglas (and womanist ethicists more generally), James Nelson, and Christine Gudorf—have not, as a rule, thoroughly engaged with or integrated these insights. This is true of Jewish ethics in particular, and in this, the discipline's foundations within modern Jewish philosophy are, on the face of it, unhelpful. Indeed, foundational Jewish philosophers like Emanuel Levinas and Eliezer Berkovits have argued the opposite: Levinas goes so far as to say that "the relationship established between lovers in [sensual pleasure],[6] fundamentally refractory to universalization, is the very contrary of the social relation. It excludes the third party, it remains intimacy, dual solitude, closed society, the supremely non-public."[7] And Berkovits claims that sex in and of itself is not only asocial but amoral as well: "Two consenting adults engaging in intercourse have little to do with any kind of ethics."[8] Scholars of Jewish ethics in particular—and I am thinking here of the important foundational work of Judith Plaskow, Rebecca Alpert, and especially Rachel Adler—who *have* engaged with this claim have not tended to be very specific or granular in their discussion of the particulars of lived sexual experience or moral development. And when more recent thinkers like Danya Ruttenberg have addressed granular details of lived sexual experience and done so with a tacit understanding of the social character of sex, they have not done so in any systematic, book-length treatment.[9]

Such a treatment is, by this point, well overdue. Here, I argue that for religious ethics, thoroughly integrating the insight that sex is part and parcel of our broader social fabric means acknowledging that it does not make sense to have a system of sexual ethics that is divorced from the ethics of our broader social lives. Furthermore, it means that the ways we shape ourselves sexually—through the sex education we receive, interpret, and disseminate, through our own sexual experiences and our secondhand experiences of and discourse on others' sexual experiences—is also a way we shape ourselves socially and morally. Someone who has learned to be a considerate, communicative sexual partner, who respects their partners' consent, desires, and safety, is likely to respect their social interlocutors' consent, desires, and safety in nonsexual situations as well. Conversely, one who does not respect these things in sexual situations is unlikely to respect them in nonsexual situations, either. Who one is in bed—not necessarily in the particulars of what turns one on but in the ways one conducts oneself toward those with whom one relates—has a great deal to do with who one is outside it.

Sexual and nonsexual social concerns never function independently from one another. Nonsexual situations are constantly infused with sexual concerns; sexual situations, conversely, do not function independently of or in isolation from nonsexual concerns. Nonsexual social situations also can be fraught in ways similar to sexual ones. While we might think of sexual interactions as mysterious and taboo breaches of normal social orders, in fact, we often carry those orders into bed with us. And, conversely, there are nonsexual situations in which the breaches of social convention we associate with sex also occur and are, in fact, expected: for example, religious rituals, theater, and the socially accepted consumption of mind-altering substances.

Sex is also a social arena in which we expect people to conform to narrow and rigid standards of perception, preference, behavior, and presentation. Sexual perceptions, desires, acts, and self-presentations that fall outside of accepted structures—in the West, usually some version of procreative, heterosexual monogamy—are coded as deviant, even unnatural, and therefore morally unacceptable. Paradoxically, though we aggressively naturalize these socially constructed standards, this is, in fact, an area where our treatment of sexual behavior comes closest to our treatment of other social behaviors: in daily, public interaction it is not acceptable to be too loud (or too quiet), too "deformed," too exposed, too needy, too Black or too brown, and so on. Generally speaking, the difference here between sex and other social interactions is one of degree rather than of kind. And yet there are modes of social interaction—particularly when it comes to matters like taste in food and drink—in which we already can admit far greater diversity in sociophysical expression of pleasure than we care to admit where sex is concerned.

In this chapter, I examine these social parallels in two steps. First, I talk about pleasure—a key component of sexual experience—as a fundamentally social phenomenon. I discuss the ways in which pleasure, especially bodily pleasure, are woven throughout our experiences as social beings; I also come to a working definition of community as both a basic unit of social relation and as a moral category that works to generate discrete interpersonal and collective duties. Second, I talk about pleasure as an idiosyncratic, diverse, and (to borrow Alasdair MacIntyre's term) polymorphous phenomenon, and I link it more broadly to diverse ways of being in community and of perceiving and interacting with one's world. I discuss the moral value of this diversity both in and of itself *and* to the communities in which it exists as a specific generator of interpersonal duties and as a source of a rich and varied range of virtues and moral disciplines.

I also examine these social parallels along two comparative axes. First, I compare sex to eating as a social phenomenon. This is an analogy with a long and star-studded history; even the classical philosophers considered the desires for sex and for food together under the rubric of "appetites." Like sex, eating is the lived and socialized practice of a basic bodily desire. Like sexual desire, people's tastes in food and drink are diverse and idiosyncratic and are formed at the intersections between some sort of biophysical givenness and various sorts of social conditioning. And, like sexual interaction, eating as an activity is simultaneously life-giving and unavoidably risky on physical, social, and psychological levels.

The second axis along which I examine these parallels, as well as the most important theoretical resource in this chapter, is through the experiences of disabled people, especially through the lenses of neurodiversity and of disability. Disability is a significant and often uncomfortably apparent way that bodies and their ways of perceiving and interacting with other bodies and their environments diverge from socially acceptable norms. It is, in other words, a stark and morally salient reminder of both the existence *and* the value of diverse ways of being in the world. In particular, I use the paradigm of neurodiversity, which was developed by autistic writer-advocates and argues that neurological differences like autism and attention deficit / hyperactivity disorder (ADHD) are valid and valuable ways of perceiving and being in the world, as a way to think about the value of diversity, both in and of itself and as a critical part of social and moral community. I link neurodivergence to sexual variation by arguing that both represent diverse ways of perceiving, processing, and responding to sensory data, and use the framework of rich and valuable social diversity articulated by the neurodiversity paradigm to argue for the more general moral worth of what I call "perceptual richness."

The social lives we live are those of bodies colliding with other bodies. Sex is one such collision; there are many others. Nevertheless, we are in the habit of assuming that the risks of sex must be treated according to separate and distinct moral categories. This is incorrect and harmful. By separating our sexual lives from the rest of our social and moral development, we neglect a critical arena in which we shape ourselves as social and moral actors. This hamstrings our ability to learn moral, respectful social conduct; it creates undiscussed social spaces in which sexual shame and sexual violence can propagate unhindered; and it creates structures through which entire classes of people have their sociosexual expression branded as deviant and unacceptable. But bringing sociosexual interaction fully into the realm of moral discussion, properly enmeshed in its broader social web, can be a first step toward correcting some of these injustices.

The Sociality of Pleasure

Empirical justice and hermeneutic competency require us to acknowledge that sex necessarily involves relationship—at the very least, to one's own body and psyche, and overwhelmingly to the bodies and psyches of others as well. Yet one of the most pernicious effects of the West's functional treatment of sex as a sui generis category is that it elides the relationality of all sex, and sexual desire has thus come to signify the apogee of individualism. The sexual urge becomes the paradigm case of selfish desire, serving as a foil against self-restraint and concern for others' needs; indeed, paradoxically, it may become so tied up in the individual body's drives that it becomes prior and even opposed to individuals' moral agency. Thus, for example, Eliezer Berkovits can make the rather bizarre claim that "two consenting adults engaging in intercourse have little to do with any kind of ethics. It is an arrangement, admittedly more civilized than rape."[10] The ethical part of sex, for Berkovits, is in the social disciplines that regulate it, which apply to but are not part of sex itself: "Jewish sexual ethics is not about sex, but about the union between a man and a woman that includes sexual fulfillment."[11] (For what it's worth, as I've discussed in chapter 1, I do agree that classical Jewish sexual ethics is, as Berkowitz puts it, "not about sex," but what I mean by that is quite different from what he does.) "Because of the tremendous power of the sexual instinct," when man (and Berkovits, I believe, really does mean "man" rather than "human") is "liberated" from the social disciplines that contain sexuality, he "falls into the thralldom of mighty impersonal forces when he liberates himself from social taboos. The sex act is not so much an act as a letting go. It is not man who acts; rather it is something that happens (the impersonal does not act) through man."[12] Sexual desire in and of itself and sexual experience in and of itself are not moral and not social in the sense that sociality necessitates morality. Rather, they are something to be contained and regulated *by* sociality and morality.

This view is pernicious rot with dangerous consequences. It is true that there is a significant component of sexual desire that is what we might call "precognitive," but sex as a lived phenomenon encompasses far more than a hormone involuntarily telling the body to increase blood flow to the genitals. That precognitive physiological response is but one component of the experience—"two consenting adults engaging in intercourse"—that Berkovits dismisses as unrelated to ethics, and nearly all of those components are deeply enmeshed in complex social relations that, in turn, are of deep moral import. (Indeed, it beggars belief that Berkovits's dismissal, as phrased, of the ethical significance of "two consenting adults engaging in intercourse" makes direct reference to the *very* ethically significant category of consent.) And even that precognitive impulse is itself conditioned over one's lifetime by a multitude of social and moral cues.

Berkovits here, then, stands as a prime example of how much Western thought tends to reduce the social activities of sex, when these are not contained by the thinker's preferred social disciplines, to solipsistic reactivity, which is unconditioned in and of itself by its environment. But this account is, quite simply, descriptively untrue. It's also dangerous and harmful. By positioning sexuality as an impersonal force, like an individual sort of gravity that has, on its own, little or to nothing to do with social interaction or moral agency—and, not incidentally, featuring the default human who experiences such a force as male—such an account enables and excuses rape and other forms of sexual violence. (Berkovits even admits as much when he says that the major difference between what he sees as undisciplined consensual sex and rape is that the former is more "civilized.") So if a sexual ethics is to responsibly account for actual human sexuality and provide some measure of genuine counterweight to sexual violence, it must begin by locating sex—not as a concept but as a real thing real people do—properly within the broader web of social actions, perceptions, and desires.

One way to do this is to think about desires for and experiences of sexual pleasure alongside desires for and experiences of other pleasures that we may more readily accept as socially shaped and morally laden. One such pleasure, to which I return as a point of comparison throughout this chapter, is that derived from eating and drinking. This pleasure has a long history of comparison to sexual pleasure, with good reason.[13] Desires to nourish oneself, like sexual desires, have a central component that is a basic precognitive urge. There's something intuitively animalistic about eating, which, if one stops to think about it, involves the act of inserting a foreign object or substance into an orifice and, hopefully, deriving pleasure from it. And yet one would be hard-pressed to think of an activity that's *more* socially regulated in more different ways—or an activity that brings public interaction, politics, and intimacy together in quite the same ways. Matters of policy, business, employment, and scholarship are discussed and decided over ritualized meals—state dinners, working lunches, professional cocktail mixers. And so are smaller matters of personal relationship—friendships might begin with coffee dates or dinner invitations or less formal instances of sharing. Romances might begin with dinner dates or drinks. We also use meals to form our more general social behavior and, indeed, as schools for our moral development—table manners, lessons about how to thank a host for the effort they have put into a meal, learning about guests' food allergies, intolerances, favorite dishes, and aversions all shape us as social and moral actors in ways that extend far beyond the table.

Importantly, in all these cases, the experience of gustatory pleasure (or displeasure) is not incidental to the character of the overall social exchange. The sensory aspects of a given experience shape its general character in significant and sustained ways. I am likelier to remember an experience fondly if I enjoyed the food that came with it; conversely, an interaction in which I found the food or drink distasteful is likelier to "leave a bad taste in my mouth" in other ways as well. The converse is also true: an experience that is unpleasant or upsetting will affect my perception and enjoyment of a taste sensation that I might otherwise like very much. Consider, for example, the common experience of overeating a much-liked food until one is sick and subsequently being "put off" that food for quite a while. (I haven't been able to stomach malted milk balls for over twenty years for precisely this reason.) Or, when one has experienced trauma, sensory stimuli linked to the traumatic event, including smells and tastes, can trigger flashbacks. Conversely, a very pleasant experience can turn an unremarkable taste into a sublime one. The food writer Nichola Fletcher recounts an acquaintance's story of savoring his last remaining morsel—a stale caraway roll—during a hiking trip for which he found he had underprovisioned: "The bursts of flavour intermittently exploding from the caraway seeds were clearly a remarkable sensation which he remembered with infectious delight."[14] And, as Fletcher conveys it, telling the story of that pleasure clearly compounded the pleasure the man took in the taste sensation and its memory; in turn, Fletcher clearly takes further pleasure in recounting the story of pleasure her acquaintance has shared with her.

So bodily, sensuous pleasure, in the form of eating and drinking, is clearly and intricately woven throughout the fabric of our broader social lives; further, this weaving tends to be accepted and acknowledged in ways that sexuality's similar interweaving is not. And yet, like taste, sexual sensation is a critical way in which we learn about our embodied existence, about the ways our particular bodies respond to stimuli and how those ways may resemble or differ from others'. Like sharing food, sexual interactions require us to attend to the particularities of others' bodies and psyches as well as those of our own. And, as with food, sexual interaction can coexist with other forms of interaction, and sexually charged thoughts and memories can and do color nonsexual experiences and interactions.

Black feminist and womanist scholars have been especially well attuned to the broad social locatedness of pleasure and the inclusion of sexual pleasure within this. As Brown Douglas articulates, "By helping Black people to affirm their very sexuality, womanist thought cultivates their potential for living out the *imago Dei* of the incarnate God, that is, being in a loving relationship with themselves and with the rest of God's creation."[15] In her pivotal essay "Uses of the Erotic," Audre Lorde writes, "the bridge which connects [the spiritual and the political] is formed by the erotic—the sensual—those physical, emotional, and psychic expressions of what is deepest and strongest and richest within each of us, being shared."[16] Taking up Lorde's thread, among others, Brown Douglas finds in the voices, bodies, and sexually frank and expressive words of Black women blues singers a model for truth telling about this connectedness and, as such, of political power: "Through their lyrics blues women did not adopt the nonsensuous norm upon which the white cultural narrative was based. By making love and desire the key for decoding the signifying message, they contested the notion that erotic sexuality is an impediment to life. Instead, they advanced sexuality as the tool for grasping life's truths. . . . They moved sex from a place of shame to a place of ultimacy. They essentially grasped the nature of sexuality itself. As blues women foregrounded sexuality, they affirmed its centrality in human existence."[17] Blues women, Brown Douglas reminds us, joyously integrated everyday sexuality—especially the doubly stigmatized sexual desires and experiences of Black women—into an art form that also interwove with multiple forms of everyday sociality. In doing so, they made their sexuality inescapably political, daring to be unashamed, sensually embodied humans within a culture that sought to deny them all of those qualities. Sexual pleasure, for the blues woman, is recreation, communication, art, and protest all at once.

Pleasure, then, or at least the *experience* of pleasure, is a deeply and inextricably social thing. And when we talk about the social units in which pleasure occurs—especially those social units we understand as carrying some kind of morally normative weight, both by setting the rules about how we may act and by encompassing those people to whom we have the most direct moral responsibilities—we often deploy the term *community* to describe it. Particularly in Jewish social ethics, community (and the Hebrew words like ḳehilah that are commonly translated as such) is a term that carries a great deal of normative weight. When Jewish ethicists, myself included, talk about sociality and especially social obligations, we're often talking about community in some sense. And, especially if we want to make a point about Jewish distinctiveness, we're likely to juxtapose some concept of community against what we perceive as the Western liberal (most often read culturally if not credally Protestant) tradition of individually centered morality.

So, particularly for a Jewish ethicist who wants a more expansive account of sexual ethics, extricating sexuality from its solipsistic pigeonhole so that one can locate it in a more communal moral context is important. I've attempted to accomplish the first part of that above. To accomplish the second part, however, I must spend some time defining just what community is, why I think it is a morally significant category, and how it links to the virtue of diverse interdependence—those qualities and structures that allow a community to comprehensively support its members without quashing those members' divergent ways of being—that I discussed in the introduction.

One of the touchstone accounts of community as a moral category in modern ethics is Michael Sandel's. Sandel distinguishes a community from within the broader category of society by asking "whether the society is itself a society of a certain kind, ordered in a certain way, such that community describes its basic structure and not merely the dispositions of persons within the structure. . . . Community must be constitutive of the shared self-understandings of the participants and embodied in their institutional arrangements, not simply an attribute of the participants' plans of life."[18] Elsewhere, Sandel further specifies that community "describes not just what [members] *have* as fellow citizens but also what they *are*, not a relationship they choose (as in a voluntary association) but an attachment they discover, not merely an attribute but a constituent of their identity."[19] So communities, for Sandel, are those societies that form around and further shape members' shared identities through structures developed with those formative purposes in mind. They are defined both in terms of affinity and in terms of formation.

While Sandel's account offers an overarching framework for defining community in moral terms, Laurie Zoloth particularizes matters, putting community in Jewish terms while sharpening its moral trajectory. She draws on her reading of classical rabbinic tradition through the philosophical lessens of Levinas, Buber, Soloveichik, and Heschel. For Zoloth, because "a self [is] a self-in-relationship" and "the issue of the obligation of the collective to the individual and the individual to the collective is critical to the understanding of what is a right act," community is "the organized collective being of the responsible self-in-relation and occurs only when all stand alert, listening both to the voice of the other person and to the command of God."[20]

Thus Zoloth roots Sandel's scaffold of affinity and formation in the language of command. If communities are formed through members' discovery of shared attributes and commitments that are constitutive of their identities, and if the community is shaped in such a way to further cultivate those attributes and commitments in common, the moral grounding of such affinity and the continuing impetus for such formation is, for Zoloth, divine command. Community occurs when "all stand alert, listening both to the voice of the other person and to the command of God"—and such command is expressed both through the explicit commands God has directly revealed through Torah and, following Levinas, through the basic moral imperative that binds a person in the moment of encounter with the other, who is the *tselem Elohim*, the "divine image." Thus affinity and formation are subsumed under the framework of covenant, which renders the bonds of affinity, the practices by which those bonds are maintained and affirmed, and the interpersonal duties that emerge from those bonds formally and metaphysically binding.

Zoloth also draws out further the reciprocal character of formation and obligation when she specifies that the moral community is formed by "selves-in-relationship." Community here is not Star Trek's Borg, in which members' particularity is assimilated and appropriated by the collective; rather, members are obligated to the collective *and* to one another in their particularity. Community, for Zoloth, is "the organized collective being of the responsible *self-in-relation*" (emphasis mine) and this entails a recognition that each self-in-relation has a distinct way-of-being that is extensively shaped by their network of relations but which those relations cannot entirely account for.

There is obviously a great deal more literature out there on the moral contours of community, but for my purposes, Sandel's categories of affinity, identity, and formation, as well as Zoloth's concept of the self-in-relation and her twofold account of divine command, offer a working definition of community that does the necessary descriptive and normative work. Thus, here, when I refer to "community," I mean "a social group organized around some sort of affinity or affinities that its members understand as somehow significantly constitutive of their individual and collective identities and which is structured in a way that promotes the further development of those characteristics that are conducive to maintaining affinity." These affinities also draw out strong moral responsibilities within the group and are generally undergirded by some sense of deontological command—in Jewish terms, divine command, which is expressed both through direct revelation and through the particular revelations of each encounter with a particular manifestation of the tselem Elohim. And when I talk about what communities must aim toward, I mean at base that they must strive toward an organized collectivity whose primary unit is the responsible *and particular* self-in-relation.

Community as a morally normative category, however, is not without its discontents, and it behooves anyone whose goals are even remotely liberationist to take these critiques seriously. The postcolonial theorist Rey Chow, beginning from a definition of community that, echoing Sandel's, is "linked to the articulation of commonality and consensus," notes that while "a community is always based on a kind of collective inclusion," nevertheless "there is no community formation without the implicit understanding of who is and who is not to be admitted."[21] Indeed, for Chow, admittance is "the principle that regulates community formation."[22] And one significant category around which admittance to a community is often based, Chow notes, is sexual conformity. Reading community formation through Freud and Fanon (here, on incest taboos), Chow highlights "the crisis-laden nature of the relationship between community and sexual difference."[23] And, historically, the paradigmatic form of sexual difference is female sexual agency (especially that of women of color). Because "any conceptualization of community is by implication a theory about reproduction, both biological and social"—and while Chow is, again, reading Freud here, I think that, inasmuch as we read reproduction of norms and affinities as a form of reproduction, this observation also applies to Sandel's definition—"female sexuality, insofar as it is the embodiment of the 'touching,' the physical intimacy that leads to such reproduction, is therefore always a locus of potential danger—of dangerous possibilities."[24]

Here, one thing Chow is asking us to attend to is that the reciprocal of affinity is exclusion. If communities are formed on the basis of shared foundations of identity, and if the structures of a community are designed to affirm, highlight, and reproduce those shared foundations, it follows that those who discover that they do not share these foundations or are judged not to share them or share them insufficiently will find themselves further and further excluded. Put more simply, if communities exist in part to draw particular people and groups in, they must necessarily cast other people and groups out. That sorting, Chow reminds us, means that communities are wielders and reproducers of power. And, inasmuch as identities and affinities are shaped by preexisting power structures, oppressive ones very much included, it is not unlikely that the affinities around which communities form and develop will, intentionally or not, reproduce preexisting oppressive power structures. Thus, for example, Miranda Joseph, in *Against the Romance of Community*, discusses the myriad ways in which explicit evocations of community in contemporary North American contexts reproduces and reinforces capitalist hegemonies. Margot Weiss, in *Techniques of Pleasure* (with which I engage in detail in chapter 5) notes the ways in which communities explicitly formed around a counterculture of sexual difference reproduce similar capitalist power dynamics. And, in the quoted essay, Chow notes the ways in which postcolonial thought (she concentrates on Fanon) can reproduce colonizers' accounts of deviant sexuality, especially female sexuality, as being fundamentally disruptive to communal cohesion, even that of explicitly postcolonial communities. Indeed, Chow ends the essay by quoting the feminist biblical scholar Mieke Bal: "The most painful sting of patriarchy is the solidarity *against* the other."[25]

Chow asks whether "female sexuality and sexual difference [could] ever be reconciled with community[.] Are these mutually exclusive events?"[26] I answer in the affirmative, but I do so with trepidation. For I suspect that to form a community that accommodates and, indeed, affirms sexual difference (as well as other forms of social difference) requires building fluidity, uncertainty, and even a certain amount of instability into the "institutional arrangements" that Sandel names. Communities must be willing to discover and rediscover changes in the affinities that constitute and define them, and so, paradoxically, one of the primary things they must not admit within their bounds is a rigid and reflexive *non*admittance. And inasmuch as communities form and focus particular moral obligations, that formation and focus must be dialectical, for, as Zoloth notes, there are obligations the collective has to the individual as well. One such obligation is the accommodation and affirmation of members' diversity, including sexual diversity. Why such is morally desirable I discuss below.

I have, throughout, been discussing sexual diversity—by which I mean, descriptively speaking, the existence of and, normatively speaking, the acknowledgment, affirmation, and accommodation of a wide variety of sexual practices, desires, and identities within a community—as though it is a good and desirable thing. I do, indeed, believe that sexual diversity *is* a good and desirable thing, but it is not necessarily self-evident, especially to those who are not part of or adjacent to the queer (in the broadest sense) community. Indeed, much of Western Christian thought has, for centuries, taken it as read that the existence of sexual variation is a form of disorder that is a consequence of the fall and ought therefore to be brought to heel through various monastic and marital disciplines. So it is important to interrogate, elucidate, and ground the contrary claim that I, here, have been similarly taking as read: that sexual diversity is a good in its own right and, indeed, a worthwhile communal discipline that is worth cultivating and sustaining.

What does sexual diversity include? Equally important, what does it stand in contradiction to? As I have already indicated, sexual diversity has both a descriptive or phenomenal sense and a prescriptive or normative sense to it; both are important to unpack. Gayle Rubin, for example, argues that "it is difficult to develop a pluralistic sexual ethics without a concept of benign sexual variation."[27] I am, as you might expect by this point, sympathetic to this argument, but it wants unpacking. In Rubin's claim, "pluralism" is a moral norm, while "sexual variation" is a descriptive statement. By applying the norm of pluralism to the observation about sexual variation, Rubin can then modify that observation with the moral descriptor "benign." But the claim, as it stands, is circular, for central to the norm of pluralism is precisely the argument that variation is benign or even actively desirable. We need to understand why a pluralistic sexual ethics is a good thing, and to do this, it may prove helpful to work in the opposite order from Rubin's claim, beginning with the descriptive observation and moving on to the explicit moral norm.

In a simple phenomenal sense, then, sexual diversity refers to any desired or practiced variation from heterosexual, "vanilla," potentially procreative PIV intercourse as practiced in private, in a monogamous marriage, without any tools or media other than the participants' own bodies and without any exchange of goods or services—anything, in other words, that falls outside of what Rubin refers to as the "charmed circle" of "sexuality that is 'good,' 'normal,' and 'natural.'"[28] Thus, it includes any sexual activity or expression among members of the LGBTQIA+ community (and, where asexual people are concerned, the deliberate nonexpression of the same); it also includes any sexual expression that might fall under the aegis of "kink," "fetish," or "paraphilia," as well as any nonmonogamous sexual expression and any masturbation. Inasmuch as society frames particular classes of people as fundamentally asexual *or* hypersexual and thus as excluded from normative sex—such as disabled people on the one hand and Black people on the other—I would consider sexual expression on the part of members of these groups as part of an expansive definition of sexual diversity; likewise, I would include any sexual expression that explicitly seeks to avoid conception. Importantly— and I address this in more detail below when I discuss the normative sense of sexual diversity and again in the next chapter when I introduce the concept of livability—there are sexual variations, such as pedophilia, that are by definition harmful. However, it is not the fact that these things are *variations* that makes them harmful; rather, it is the fact that their expression by definition harms others.

Descriptively speaking, sexual diversity also accounts for the particulars of any given sexual encounter—the physical movements and sensations, the aesthetics, the emotions involved, and the reasons for engaging in that particular act. Ethicists have an unfortunate habit of speaking of sex—or "good" sex, anyway—in lofty, aspirational terms: the physical and spiritual union of committed partners, the human sharing in divine creativity, the two becoming one, and so on. This image of choreographed perfection is reproduced in popular culture—sex scenes in movies and television shows feature toned bodies, with skin glowing in perfect lamplight, moving in visually pleasing synchrony while emitting rhythmic and consonant moans. There is a conspicuous absence of fumbles or fluids of any kind. (It was notable, for example, that in a 2013 sex scene between two women that otherwise featured many of these idealized tropes, the Canadian urban fantasy series *Lost Girl* showed one of the women with conspicuously wet fingers.)[29] Even in sex comedies, the bodies are perfect (unless the character is meant to be considered sexually disgusting, in which case their imperfections are wildly exaggerated), and the screams and fumbles are carried out with perfect comic timing.

But the actual practice of sex, by ordinary people, is not so lofty, so beautifully synchronous. Real sex, even "good" sex, is carnivalesque, even grotesque. Real sex involves fluids, farts, jiggling, grunting, adjustments of position, arms falling asleep, and accidental pinching or pulling of hair. It involves small talk, fumbling, sometimes-tedious negotiation—"Here?" "No, up to the left a bit . . . no, down!"—and the making of a vast number of frankly ridiculous faces. It is often peppered with distractions, jokes, and mundane asides. Nor is any given instance of it necessarily the result of simultaneous and overwhelming love or even lust. Levels of desire between partners are hardly ever in perfect synchrony, and even within a long-term, committed relationship, one partner may freely consent to sex to keep another partner happy, even if they themselves are not particularly interested. People may have sex—whether by themselves or with a partner or partners—out of boredom, as a means of stress relief, as part of paid work, or for any number of other reasons that may have, in the moment, little or nothing to do with regnant portraits of sex as the ritual that confirms some picture of love and duty between two committed romantic partners.

In a normative sense, sexual diversity as a category considers the above phenomenal description and concludes that, in light of the existence of such a range of sexual expression, it is problematic in the extreme to figure one particular version of heterosexual monogamy, enacted for the purposes of one particular vision of love and duty, and choreographed just so, as the default or norm. If there is any default, this normative sense of the term argues, it *is* variation. Indeed, the normative sense of sexual diversity will have done one critical part of its work when that vision of heterosexual monogamy no longer excludes itself from the phenomenal description of sexual diversity and takes its place as one sort of expression among many—not such that queer identities and experiences become flattened, default, "just like everyone else," but such that heterosexual monogamy too is productively destabilized and subject to questioning and that there is no default.

Sexual diversity, thus, bursts open Gayle Rubin's "charmed circle" and stands in opposition to what Adrienne Rich classically described as "compulsory heterosexuality," in which heterosexual intercourse is naturalized and becomes default, nonspecific, and the only "normal" possibility for sexual expression and for the social and economic structures built around that scaffolding. Through the lens of compulsory heterosexuality, writes Rich, "lesbian"—though we can easily expand this to the more general "queer"— "experience is perceived on a scale ranging from deviant to abhorrent, or simply rendered invisible."[30] Against this, sexual diversity as a normative category seeks to dislodge a very narrow version of heterosexual intercourse from its place as default and instead to situate it as one possibility among many. The normative sense of sexual diversity goes further, then, in that it claims that this range of sexual variations not only exists but is actually desirable for its own sake.

Importantly, this normative sense of sexual diversity does *not* claim that any given act that may fall within the descriptive sense of sexual diversity is good or desirable simply or only because it is different. Sexual diversity in its normative sense is not morally anarchic. Any sexual expression or act that is harmful or oppressive to others is morally wrong, regardless of whether that act is included in the descriptive sense of sexual diversity. Indeed, part of the moral critique of compulsory heterosexuality is precisely that it is harmful or oppressive to others; disrupting compulsory heterosexuality is thus morally desirable. But this disruption, while *necessary* to the normative sense of sexual diversity, is far from sufficient. A morally desirable diversity does not merely exchange some harms or oppressions for others but works to reduce harm and oppression across the board. Communities have collective duties toward their members' well-being. This includes clarifying the limits of acceptable conduct and ensuring to the best of their abilities that malefactors are unable to use a commitment to sexual diversity as a cover or excuse for predatory behavior—as, for example, the musician and media personality Jian Ghomeshi did when he characterized alleged violent sexual assaults against multiple female partners merely as kinky sex.[31] Individuals and communities also need to accept that, for those who have had traumatic experiences linked to a given activity, that activity may remain forever tainted for them. To the extent, however, that sexually diverse or alternative communities reproduce harmful power dynamics found *within* the "charmed circle"—a phenomenon I explore in greater detail in chapter 5—these should be understood not as indictments of sexual diversity as such but instead as indicting a broader systematic problem that infuses all social structures.

Sexual diversity, then, overlaps with queerness in the broadest sense of that term, in that it destabilizes systems of compulsory heterosexuality. But it expands far beyond the queer community in the narrower sense—a married, monogamous couple consisting of two cisgender heterosexuals, as I have discussed above, participates in sexual diversity in some sense if they so much as employ birth control, let alone if they engage in the occasional act of light bondage.

Nevertheless, the queer community, especially as we have become increasingly visible in recent decades, stands in many ways as an example par excellence of the normative power of sexual diversity. The queer community's very existence forces us to take as given the descriptive sense of sexual diversity and to center the conversation squarely on the normative sense of the same. Queers undeniably exist, and this existence remains threatening to significant numbers of people. It is useful to understand why this is. And, in fact, one reason queer sexuality is threatening is that it forces us to confront the fact that sexual desires, practices, and identities are far more diverse and fluid than can be easily fitted into neat and tractable categories. The ability to taxonomize is the ability to contain and control, and so queer sexuality represents that sexuality that is beyond reliable containment and control.

It is for this reason, among others, that at least some versions of virtue ethics are highly congenial to a friendly analysis of queer sexuality. Virtues can tend toward unruliness: a tumbling multitude of ever-reproducing and likely redundant qualities, dispositions, and signifiers that threaten to spill out of the boundaries of neatly ordered moral categories (even though, ironically enough, the most prominent systems of virtue ethics have stressed containment, discipline, and order!). And yet it is precisely this unruliness, this threatened redundancy, this fluidity, that allows virtue ethics to better account for what Alasdair MacIntyre has called "the polymorphous character of pleasure" and, in turn, to also account for the multifarious character of queer sexuality.[32]

Queer sexuality, then, demonstrates that sexual diversity *is*. I argue further that sexual diversity, as a form of social diversity, is not only a thing that is and must be accounted for but is also morally desirable in its own right. In addition to queer theory, I draw here on MacIntyre's concept of the polymorphous character of pleasure, as well as the neurodiversity paradigm, which argues that such neurological differences as autism, ADHD, dyslexia, and Tourette's syndrome are in fact invaluable variations within the universe of human cognition.

Pleasure and Its Variations and Valences

In his extensive critique of classic Enlightenment-era utilitarianism in *After Virtue*, MacIntyre took aim at the usefulness of "pleasure" as a utilitarian metric by pointing to its "polymorphous character."[33] Contra Mill and, before him, Bentham, MacIntyre claims that pleasure and the related, though far broader category of happiness "[are] *not* [u]nitary, simple notion[s] and cannot provide us with a criterion for making our key choices."[34] Rather, he asserts, pleasures—much, one might say, like virtues[35]—are multifarious and irreducible to one another; they aren't even comparable to one another according to a single standard:

> For there are too many different kinds of enjoyable activity, too many different modes in which happiness is achieved. And pleasure or happiness are not states of mind for the production of which these activities and models are merely alternative means. The pleasure-of-drinking-Guinness is not the pleasure-of-swimming-at-Crane's-Beach, and the swimming and the drinking are not two different means for providing the same end-state. The happiness which belongs peculiarly to the way of life of the cloister is not the same happiness as that which belongs peculiarly to the military life. For different pleasures and different happinesses are to a large degree incommensurable:

there are no scales of quantity or quality on which to weigh them. Consequently appeal to the criteria of pleasure will not tell me whether to drink or swim and appeal to those of happiness cannot decide for me between the life of a monk and that of a soldier.[36]

I do not agree with MacIntyre's claim that, because pleasures are multifarious and irreducible, it is therefore impossible to use them as sources for moral reasoning. Indeed, as I argue throughout and am about to argue quite specifically, pleasures are incredibly important data for such. What MacIntyre is quite correct about, however, is that pleasure as a general concept is polymorphous and irreducible. Pleasures are also protean: the pleasure-of-drinking-Guinness outdoors with friends on a spring afternoon while discussing a particularly thorny bit of text is not the same as the pleasure-of-drinking-Guinness by oneself in a comfortable chair with a good book. Furthermore, each time one experiences a particular instantiation of the pleasure-of-drinking-Guinness, memories and associations from that instantiation will accrue to one's lifetime experience of the overall pleasure-of-drinking-Guinness, such that even if I drank Guinness two days in a row, in the same chair, with the same book, the second pleasure would be different from the first because it now evoked the memories of the first.

Further, not only is the pleasure-of-drinking-Guinness different from the pleasure-of-swimming-at-Crane's-Beach, but these experiences vary from person to person as to how pleasurable one will find them or even whether one will find the same thing pleasurable at all. Indeed, the very examples he chooses—beer, with its bitter flavor and intoxicating properties, and swimming, an acquired skill and a risk activity—are prime examples of things that some people find highly pleasurable and others find deeply repugnant. The fact that some people enjoy the bitter flavors of beer or the unmooring sensation of being swept along by a body of water—or the tongue-burning pain of habanero chiles or the ache of quadriceps flooded with lactic acid after a hard run or the sting of a riding crop on their buttocks—while others find these sensations unpleasant or repulsive reminds us that pleasure is varied and irreducible not only from experience to experience and from time to time but also from person to person.

If pleasure cannot be standardized or reduced, there can be, therefore, no normative definition of pleasure beyond "that sensation which some person at some point enjoys." One reason for this is that, as we have discussed, pleasure is protean, and enjoyment is necessarily a moving target. I find things pleasurable now that I found deeply unpleasant five years ago, and there are things I found pleasurable years ago that I find unpleasant (or merely unremarkable) now. What is pleasurable varies between people, and it also varies throughout a person's lifetime because, again, past experiences condition future ones such that sensations become heavily laden with memory and meaning. The act of deciding what will be pleasurable thus becomes an ongoing process of interpretation.

Again, this is something we understand more intuitively with food and drink, to the point that we even have a name for one such evolution—that of the "acquired taste." To return once more to the example of beer: beer is, as we have discussed, usually mildly to bracingly bitter, and many people who first taste it (myself included) find the bitterness unpleasant. But beer drinking is quite often an important social ritual, and the beverage delivers other sensations that might be less immediately repulsive (cold temperature, carbonation, sweeter or richer flavors from malt, and so on), so there are often reasons why those of us who find beer repulsive on first encounter keep trying it again and again until one day, we find that we tolerate or even enjoy the bitterness. And even this process of "acquiring tastes" is not uniform for all people. Some people genuinely enjoy bitter flavors almost immediately and do not need repeated exposure to acclimate. And even tastes toward which we are already predisposed in some way can be influenced by experience and environment.

Sexual tastes are similarly subject to processes of ongoing interpretation, and they are similarly mediated by and evolve according to our continually accruing experiences of socially located sexuality. This is not to say that sexual tastes are infinitely mutable, and it is certainly not to say that we can unilaterally decide, "Well, I want to enjoy *this* and not that, so I'll engineer my social experiences to change things." Contrary both to the homophobic claim that "deviant" sexual preferences can be "corrected" through therapy *and* to the naive and reductionist "born-this-way-ism" that characterizes certain spheres within gay-rights activism, sexual desires have aspects that are "given" in some way and not open to being deliberately shaped in a given direction; these and other interconnected aspects *are*, however, subject to constant subtle mediation and shaping by our lived individual and communal experiences.

Here, the comparison to gustatory tastes breaks down slightly, for some research indicates that, at least up to a certain point, even strong dislikes for certain foods can be modified through repeated encounters with minute quantities of the food.[37] Sexual preferences cannot always be modified so directly, perhaps in part because, even more so than tastes in food and drink, people are liable to experience particular sexual desires as being significantly constitutive of their identities. In this way, for example, sexual minorities form communities based on affinities that most members consider inextricable from their identities; indeed, members of LGBTQIA+ and kink communities frequently use the language of "discovery" instead of or in addition to the language of choice to describe those aspects of their identities. Furthermore, the systematic (rather than circumstantial) denial of opportunities for sexual fulfillment in ways that are coherent with one's self-understanding is frequently experienced as deeply destructive to one's sense of self. At the same time, however, sexual preferences, especially those that one experiences, at least initially, as less constitutive of identity *are* sometimes modifiable with experience—consider the (anecdotally) common case of someone with "vanilla" sexual tastes engaging in bondage play for the sake of a partner who enjoys it and, over time, coming to enjoy that play themselves. Or, conversely, a practice someone once enjoyed may become unpleasant or even triggering if it becomes associated with a traumatic experience.

It is important to understand that sexual fulfillment is not a one-size-fits-all proposition. Even the parts of our sexual makeup that are precognitive and pre-social exhibit variation, and sex's fundamentally social character means that no two persons' sexual selves will be formed by precisely the same constellation of relationships and other social influences. The range of preferred sexual expression formed by these disparate variables—both social and precognitive or pre-social—is vast. This is surely the case for the publicly visible aspects of a person's sexuality: heterosexual monogamy may be satisfying and sufficient for one person, difficult but workable for another, and utterly stultifying for a third. And even within a relationship model that is generally agreeable to its participants, variation persists and even expands. One member of a couple may require a vibrator to achieve orgasm, while the other requires role-play or pornography to fully immerse themselves in the sexual encounter.

Variation occurs not only in sexual preferences themselves but in the extent to which the opportunity to pursue a given preference is necessary for overall fulfillment. People may have several preferences that an opportunity to pursue would be very nice indeed but that they could as happily do without, especially if by doing without those preferences they gained something equally or more valuable. Someone may very much enjoy tying up a sexual partner but consider it well worth depriving themselves of that preference for the sake of maintaining a comfortable and humane relationship with a particular partner for whom bondage, even when consensual, evokes traumatic memories. For a different person, however, practicing BDSM may be so integral to sexual fulfillment that they would be unable to thrive in a relationship with someone who was unwilling or unable to participate or to allow them to practice BDSM outside the relationship.

In cases where a particular preference exists but is not essential for sexual fulfillment, someone could probably exist comfortably within a system of sociosexual ethics that is more narrow and restrictive. In cases where a particular sexual preference is necessary for sexual fulfillment, however, a person with a sexuality that deviates from prescribed norms will find that restrictive system of sexual ethics unlivable. As both psychological data and the lived experience of sexual minority communities indicate, forcing someone into a role incongruous with their sexual orientation can cause severe psychological harm. The damage done to lesbian, gay, and bisexual people by "conversion therapy" programs is perhaps the clearest demonstration of this. The harm done by being forced into incongruous roles—or by not being allowed into any role at all—is clearly a risk people take into consideration in the course of their sexual decision-making. It is also a risk that ethicists and community leaders ought to take seriously.

Sexual Diversity and Neurodiversity

If people's experiences of sexual interest and sexual pleasure are so diverse as to seriously complicate any single standard of sexual normalcy, what moral frameworks *can* account for this diversity? One possibility comes from the neurodiversity movement.

The term *neurodiversity* is generally credited to the sociologist Judy Singer, who coined it in response to both an increasing recognition of autism as a spectrum of neurological, behavioral, and perceptual differences rather than a discrete and catastrophic disorder and to the increased visibility of autistic self-advocates who identified strongly with and took pride in those differences. As Singer writes, "Neurodiversity takes postmodern fragmentation one step further. Just as the postmodern era sees every once too solid belief melt into air, even our most taken-for-granted assumptions—that we all more or less see, feel, touch, hear, smell, and sort information, in more or less the same way (unless visibly disabled)—are being dissolved."[38]

The neurodiversity paradigm argues that autism, ADHD, and other neurodivergences not only represent alternative ways of processing information and social relations but that those differences are valuable in and of themselves. As the journalist Harvey Blume wrote, "Neurodiversity may be every bit as crucial for the human race as biodiversity is for life in general. Who can say what form of wiring will prove best at any given moment?"[39] Years earlier, Singer herself, given an assignment by her rabbi to rewrite the Ten Commandments, articulated the underlying commitment to diversity of all kinds with startling poetic and moral force: "Honor diversity, lest thou endeth up like unto the cactus of the desert."[40] Different ways of processing information offer communities a broader range of perspectives and tools for navigating, managing, and adapting to a variety of scenarios. So, in addition to doing unforgivable violence to neurodivergent members by forcing them to conform to neurotypical expectations or eliminating them entirely, communities harm themselves by failing to support and appreciate the perspectival richness those members offer.

One thing about a neurodiversity paradigm that is particularly congenial for thinking about sexual diversity is that neurodivergence deals in large part with differences in the way people process sensory input. For example, a sound that is pleasant to one neurotypical person and unpleasant to another might, for an autistic person, be so overwhelming as to make it difficult or impossible to conduct regular activities. For someone with ADHD,[41] similarly (and in both cases I write from my own experience), sounds that a neurotypical person might experience as mildly irritating background noise can render focusing on a basic task infernally difficult. Conversely, other, chosen sounds can occupy the ADHD brain's near-constant need for external stimuli enough to permit sustained focus. (In fact, listening to Wendy Carlos's rendition of Bach's Sinfonia to Cantata no. 29 is helping me focus sufficiently to draft this very paragraph.)

Indeed, these perceptual differences often cross over into sexuality itself. As Rachel Groner notes, "Certain aspects of [autism spectrum disorder]—in particular, an intolerance for being touched that some autistic people experience—make some conventional sexual acts unpleasant or undesirable and thus necessitate alternative modes of sexual and sensual expression."[42] Groner further notes that "some [autistic] individuals with heightened or diminished sensory abilities have to adjust normative sexual activities for their bodies,"[43] as they may experience the same activity in very different ways. But, she adds, this need for adjustment is not alien to neurotypicals; it is "a process that NT people also engage in, albeit in less conscious ways."[44] Neurodivergent people draw stark attention to the vast range of ways it is possible for someone to process and experience sensory input, but this variety, and the need to adjust for it, is far from being the exclusive preserve of "deviants." Rather, it is exactly variety that is the norm.

One thing I am therefore arguing is that by juxtaposing sexual diversity with neurodiversity, we can understand sexuality as socialized *perception*. Sexuality deals with the ways we react to sensory data and integrate them into our social interactions, which in turn conditions and reconditions our ongoing interpretations both of those data and of the interactions during which they occur. Different people react to, process, and integrate the sensory data associated with sexuality differently than others, and so they will perceive different sensory data as more pleasurable than others. And, much as neurodiversity highlights and celebrates the wide range of ways humans respond to and integrate sensory stimuli more broadly, a normative account of sexual diversity will highlight and celebrate the wide range of ways humans respond to sexual sensations as one part of the range of human sensory response and interpretation.

The Moral Case for Sexual Diversity: Building Livable, Socially Adaptable Communities

What the cases of sexual diversity and neurodiversity should both demonstrate is that significant perceptual variation exists among and within human communities and that there is usually something about this variation that is intrinsic to one's sense of self and difficult or impossible to predictably and substantially modify without doing serious harm. What neurodiversity should further elucidate is that these perceptual variations are valuable in and of themselves. The neurodiversity paradigm, as with many parts of the disability movement more broadly, argues that not only should neurodivergent and otherwise disabled people be respected and accepted as they already are—we might say *bedi'avad*, or "after the fact"—without pressure to be "fixed" or "cured" but that divergent minds and bodies are valuable in and of themselves, *l'khathilah*, or "to begin with."[45] Different kinds of embodiment contribute to the richness of human experience and offer diverse ways of perceiving and responding to all kinds of sensory and conceptual input. There are, in short, as many valuable variations of ways of being as there are individual beings.

How might we integrate this diversity into a communal moral framework and move from the irreducible "is" of these diversities to the "ought" of affirming and accommodating them in a way that is fully integrated into our common moral lives? Jewish moral and philosophical traditions do not lack for accounts of the moral value of relationship or of difference. Martin Buber emphasized the importance of the uniqueness of beings within an intersubjective, "I-Thou" relation.[46] Emmanuel Levinas, classically, argued that it is precisely the other's alterity and vulnerability that creates the moral duties from which all relations subsequently proceed.[47] What these accounts capture in one way or another is that communal moral duties arise through acts of relation to an other. And, to the extent that we derive our moral responsibilities toward each other through our interpersonal relationships, relating specifically *across difference* is a critical component of that fundamental derivation.

This also means that diversity and vulnerability are intimately linked, and both have the force of moral command. As Laurie Zoloth puts it, "The vulnerability of the face imposed its own demands. . . . The vulnerability recalled the command not to kill, and alterity recalled respect for difference."[48] And we certainly have myriad evidence that it is often precisely difference that makes one vulnerable. In the specific cases I discuss here, unfortunately, another trait common to both neurodivergent people and people whose sexual divergence is publicly known is the stigma associated with both states. The specifics of the stigma differ: neurodivergent people (if their neurodivergence is recognized at all) are variously cast as nonagents, objects of pity or remote disgust, or malingerers and are often desexualized. Sexual "deviants," by contrast, are often cast as willful miscreants, selfish consumers, or victims of sexual malfeasance and are often reduced to little more than their sexuality. Thus, sex, as Gayle Rubin reminds us, "is a vector of oppression. The system of sexual oppression cuts across other modes of social inequality, sorting out individuals and groups according to its own intrinsic dynamics."[49] One aspect of this system is exclusion from "legitimate" sexual expression if one perceives the world "wrong."

Thus, perhaps in this relation between alterity, vulnerability, and moral obligation, we can begin to flesh out why perceptual diversity is valuable to *everyone*. One whose divergent perceptions cash out in social and behavioral divergences and who has been done violence on that account is, to begin with, a vulnerable other, the encounter with whom generates moral duties. This is all the more true and apparent for those who experience oppression, especially in the face of oppressive social structures that frame alterity as grounds for *negating* moral obligation toward the one who diverges. But the intimate link between divergence, vulnerability, and moral obligation also affects the way that vulnerable, divergent others shape themselves in relation to their divergence and their vulnerability, especially to those structures that punish it. Perceptual differences engender different and valuable techniques of self, what Susan Wendell, referring to disabled and chronically ill people's experiences, calls "valuable *ways of being*."[50] Perceptual differences reveal in day-to-day interactions and communications different aspects of meaning, different ways that a given action might harm or help, and one who lives with such perceptual differences will shape oneself morally according to those different moral aspects of interaction that they discover. And it is only through allowing those differences to flourish, and through interacting across all our differences, that we can begin to fulfill the myriad social and relational duties that our encounters bring into being. As Alison Kafer puts it (again, speaking of disability), "To eliminate disability"—which is, among other things, a kind of perceptual divergence—"is to eliminate the possibility of discovering alternative ways of being in the world, to foreclose the possibility of recognizing and valuing our interdependence."[51]

If—to return to the complaint I discussed at the beginning of this section—the virtues are "an unruly lot," then not merely accommodating but actively affirming difference shows us precisely the value of that unruliness. And sexual divergence is very much included here. For acknowledging different ways of perceiving sexual sensation, and acknowledging that those divergences may not always follow a predictable logic, reminds us just how impossible it is to contain the other. We must not presume. We must ask. We must keep asking and listening and responding. And we must be mindful always of that other's vulnerability, as well as of our own, and of the unpredictable character of just how any of us might be vulnerable.

I thus return to what I referred to above as "perspectival richness." For different ways of perceiving and acting in the world also generate different ways of navigating that world, navigating oneself and one's place in it, and shaping oneself as a moral actor in relation to other, different, and differently vulnerable moral actors. Just as neurodivergent members contribute different and valuable perspectives and social and moral techniques to their communities, so, too, do sexually divergent members contribute different and valuable perspectives and social and moral techniques. Navigating sexual difference—and navigating the stigma sexual difference has carried and often continues to carry—elucidates different moral facets of sociosexual encounters that sexually divergent members have had to learn to manage. Those management strategies, though, may prove invaluable to all members of a community, sexually typical and sexually divergent alike.

3. RISKY BUSINESS

Why Risk Is Inherent in Sociality

I REMEMBER ONE DAY, I think during the summer I turned nine, I had a school friend over to play. "Estelle" was tall, attractive, and popular, and I very much wanted to impress her, but I also felt comfortable enough to engage in the sort of uninhibited silliness that is developmentally appropriate for children of that age. I don't remember whether Estelle was bothered by my behavior, but I do remember that after we dropped her off at her house that afternoon, my father turned to me and said something like, "Estelle is a very good friend. You should be careful not to lose her." The conversation that followed made it clear that this "carefulness" meant "you should be careful to avoid behaving as you did today if you don't want to scare her off."

I learned quite clearly that day that social interaction—even the "innocent" play of children—is an inherently risky enterprise. You tried to make friends, at least in part, to cultivate a group of people with whom you could be some uninhibited version of yourself, yet, ironically, the making of friends required a performance that called for significant self-inhibition. The development of friendships required careful calculation as to how much disinhibition to allow oneself, at what stage of the relationship, and during which moments within it. I saw that there were people who could navigate these calculations with a careless ease, one that seemed wholly alien to me. But I badly wanted to be included in such a group, and I wanted that group to be "popular," at that, since I liked (and still like) being admired and feared a bit more than is probably healthy. So I learned to approximate that apparent ease as best I could, even though most of my actions came with a frisson of hesitation and anxiety.

I share this anecdote because it reveals the ways in which even the most innocent sorts of social interaction—two young children playing together, supervised by a parent—can harbor significant social-emotional risks. Such interactions call up questions of self-revelation and self-policing, of identity, social position, and rejection, questions that are also deeply and specifically salient to sexual interaction.

Why is risk the pivot of this book? First, risk is entangled with and in several ways central to the virtues of empirical justice, hermeneutic competency, wise risk management, and diverse interdependence that I argue the ways of thinking and reading I demonstrate here cultivate. Second, we specifically tend to separate sex from the rest of sociality on the basis of risk. For while risk is often deployed as a justification for restrictive and socially disconnected systems of sexual ethics, there are, in fact, myriad nonsexual situations in which explicit or tacit rules must be negotiated at great emotional or physical risk. There are, similarly, nonsexual situations in which the vagaries of the porous and appetitive body must be publicly negotiated.

In this chapter, I discuss the risks inherent in *all* forms of social interaction—not just sex. Circling back to the value of diversity and to the analytical lenses of neurodivergence and disability, as I discussed in the previous chapter, I note that marginalized actors—including and especially those labeled as "deviant" by narrow and restrictive social structures—offer us a range of virtues that may be particularly well suited to managing that inherent social risk. Also, for many disabled people, the physical, psychological, and social risks inherent in day-to-day interaction are heightened to the point where it becomes impossible for the person who experiences those risks to ignore or interpret them away, as those of us who are able-bodied often do.

I use crip theory, whose contours as a field are most clearly articulated by Robert McRuer and Carrie Sandhal and which makes an explicit point of centering the lived experiences and self-accounting of disabled people and which applies many of the analytical and theoretical categories of queer theory to understanding those disabled experiences, as a way to think through social risk, its moral value, and the moral techniques people use to manage those risks.[1] Crip theory argues, at base, that systems of compulsory heterosexuality and compulsory able-bodiedness delineate a normative way of being in the world that is, among other things, free from risk. Crip experience, like queer experience, stands as stark testimony as to the impossibility of that way of being. It positions acknowledging, embracing, and negotiating risk as a moral and political action that fundamentally challenges these impossible yet compulsory structures. These moral techniques of acknowledgment, navigation, and negotiation, I argue, are techniques all of us—queer or not, disabled or not—would do well to cultivate, both in terms of our sexual lives and in terms of our social lives more generally.

From this, I draw out two key concepts for thinking about and managing social risk that will be operative in the remaining chapters of the book: livability and discernment. Livability, which I define as a state of dynamic balance among one's own needs and desires, the needs and desires of individual others with whom one interacts, and the basic structures of the social orders in which one lives, such that flourishing is accessible to everyone and that no one experiences unbearable hardship, describes the ultimate and continuing goal of risk management. Discernment, which I define as the capacity to observe, analyze, weigh, and make careful judgments concerning information related to risks and goods as they may affect oneself and others, is a key virtue for the ongoing practice of risk management.

Finally, I transition from part I of the book, which deals with theoretical and conceptual groundings, to part II, which applies the groundings to case studies that put contemporary problems in dialogue with classical rabbinic texts, by briefly exploring the ins and outs of social risk as they appear in the story of Rabbi Yoḥanan and Resh Laḳish in Bavli Bava Metsia 84a–b. I read the story as a poignant reminder both of the deeply risky character of any intimate social interaction, sexual or otherwise, and of the often inseparable relationship between social risk and livability.

The Risks of Sociality

Sex is dangerous—in case we require reminding on that point. Sexual interaction opens us up to risks of infection, violence, and, if we are in possession of functional ovaries and a uterus, pregnancy. And it opens us up to social and psychological risks as well. Sex can leave us feeling violated, exposed, and worthless. It can leave us feeling stupid and ridiculous. It can open us up to feelings of loss and rejection when we end an intimate relationship or when we pursue the beginning of such a relationship and are rebuffed.

So far, so good. It would be foolish to argue that sex is not risky. And so it is in part because of these risks that we are exhorted to restrict sex to certain narrow contexts. Sex, we are told, is dangerous, and the only way to mitigate that danger is to limit its expression to marriage or, at the very least, to long-term monogamous relationships. And it is because of the dangers of sex that certain populations we have deemed vulnerable—teenagers, the elderly, the disabled—should avoid it (assuming, that is, we even acknowledge them as sexual beings).

It is here, though, that the argument begins to break down. For while sex is risky, it is not the only risky thing any of us do on a regular basis, and if we were to apply this logic consistently, many of us would find ourselves leading severely curtailed lives. Even bracketing the fact that these restrictions do not eliminate the risks of sex (being married, for example, is hardly a prophylactic against intimate partner violence, although it seems to be a remarkably effective means of disguising it), what these voices miss is that the general types of risk I have said are associated with sex are not associated with sex *exclusively*. Sex is *not* the only way to spread or contract infection. It is *not* the only way one can be a victim of violence—even, paradoxically, sexual violence, since, as feminist scholars and activists have noted repeatedly, sexual assault and sexual harassment are primarily matters of power in which sex is a means rather than an end and that people are often subjected to such behavior in explicitly nonsexual circumstances. Sex is *not* the only way one can be exploited, and it is *not* the only social context in which one can feel violated, exposed, worthless, or rejected. It is, however, with the exception of the consumption of mind-altering substances, the *only* form of social interaction from which entire classes of people are exhorted to abstain and whose expression everyone is exhorted to restrict severely on the basis of those risks.

At this point, I want to clarify what I mean by the category of risk and to distinguish it from some other related yet distinct categories that are of moral import here. First, it should be noted that *risk studies* can denote a range of interdisciplinary areas of study across the social sciences, including the cultural theory of risk first elaborated by Mary Douglas and Aaron Wildavsky, which maintains that risk tolerance is organized according to a community or subcommunity's levels of hierarchy ("grid") and collectivity ("group").[2] There are also more psychologically or economically inflected

models of risk perception, as well as interdisciplinary models like the social
amplification of risk framework, which argues that "hazards interact with
psychological, social, institutional, and cultural processes in ways that may
amplify or attenuate public responses to the risk or risk event."[3] Closer to
my own field, bioethicists work with a range of concepts around risk and
engage a number of active problems regarding risk perception, with particular attention to its relationship to questions of informed consent and
medical decision-making on the parts of patients and clinicians alike.[4] In
the field of Jewish bioethics in particular, Benjamin Freedman has used the
halakhic categories of *tsa'ar*, or "pain," and *sakanah*, or "danger," to distinguish between the risk of experiencing suffering and the risk of sustaining
harm—the latter of which the medical provider is the contingent authority regarding and the former of which the patient is the *ultimate* authority
regarding.[5]

My own working understanding of risk draws on all these areas to varying degrees but does not fit squarely within any one of them. For me, risk is
a moral category—or, more precisely, it is a phenomenon whose perceived
contours shape individuals and communities as moral agents. Indeed, risk
is one of the most morally salient phenomena for our development as moral
agents because it is, in one way or another, ubiquitous. Along these lines, my
account shares significant common ground with some of the major concepts
in Sharon Welch's *A Feminist Ethic of Risk*. Welch, drawing on the work of
Black feminist and womanist scholars, writers, and activists, emphasizes
the importance of "[acknowledging] the costs of our attempts to do good."
Welch's sources "call us to an ethic of risk, realizing that victories are always
partial, their value resident in the matrix of possibilities created."[6] An ethic
of risk, for Welch, means acting to repair the world in full recognition of
its brokenness and one's own risk of failure. It means taking contingent,
imperfect actions that, bit by bit, build the conditions necessary for further
justice work. Such action shapes individuals and communities in ways that
are conducive to building such conditions.

My account of risk is also similar to that implied by the concept of "dignity of risk," a term coined in 1972 by Robert Perske regarding the rights of
intellectually disabled people, which has since become a core tenet of the
independent living movement as well as of broader disability rights activism.[7]
According to this framework, risk is not only a normal and unavoidable part

of life, but insulating a given class of persons from normal risk more so than others constitutes discrimination and moral and psychic harm. To have the opportunity to respond to risk—by which, at the most fundamental level I mean *uncertainty of outcome*—is a critical part of how one develops as an agent who can respond to other agents with care and respect. While communities can and should come to some form of consensus regarding tolerable and intolerable levels of risk in any given context, substantially denying this basic opportunity to anyone, especially on the basis of divergence from a regnant norm, *in and of itself* constitutes harm regardless of further consequences.

At this point, I must distinguish the phenomenon of *damage* and the sensation of *hurt* or *pain* from the phenomena of *harm* and *suffering* and distinguish all of these from the phenomenon of *risk*. By damage, I mean a rupture of some aspect of someone or something's structural integrity, whether that be somatic, psychological, social, or material. By hurt or pain, I mean a sensation, often though not always intense relative to one's baseline level of sensation, that indicates that some kind of damage has occurred. Note that at this point I have not yet introduced any normative qualifiers. All other things being equal, one may wish to avoid damage, pain, or hurt but not always. For example, often, to remedy damage one must first do further damage: removing parts of a building to remodel it, say, or removing decayed parts of a tooth to fill it. And sometimes, as I discussed in chapter 2, people enjoy painful sensations. This is a book about sex, so BDSM—about which, more in chapter 5—is an obvious example, but it is not the only one, as anyone who enjoys running marathons, watching horror movies, or eating very hot chiles can easily confirm. The categories of harm and suffering, which always involve damage but are not coextensive with it, add these normative qualifications. By harm, I mean undesirable damage to a person's somatic, psychological, material, or social being that negatively affects their or others' flourishing; by suffering, I mean the painful sensation or experience of harm. Finally, by risk, I mean the relative probability that some unpleasant or harmful outcome may occur, either along with or instead of some neutral or beneficial outcome.

Thus, when I argue, as I do throughout, that a moral baseline for acceptable social activity, sexual and otherwise, is that it does not harm others, I am *not* saying that such activity must be free of the risk of harm, nor am I saying it must never involve hurt or pain. There is an important and valid ongoing process of discernment to engage in as to what constitutes a morally acceptable threshold of risk for an individual or a community to shoulder, but levels of risk are not the same things as intrinsic harms. I often wonder, for example, whether I have any authority to criticize American football as it is currently played, even though we are beginning to grasp the appalling rates of repeated head trauma associated with it, given that my sport of choice, equestrianism, is statistically one of the riskiest sports out there.[8] But even though equestrianism involves a relatively high risk of severe injury, falling off and sustaining a concussion or breaking a rib is not baked into the objective of any equestrian sport in the same way that repeatedly ramming one's head into other players at high speed, thus doing regular, cumulative, concussive harm, is part and parcel of the normal course of a football game, even one in which nothing goes awry. Similarly, the practice of telling jokes may risk social or psychological harm to others, and, indeed, the risks of harm and benefit in humor are often inseparable, since some of the most powerful and funniest humor may deal with very dark, painful, and potentially harmful subject matter. Racist, sexist, or otherwise bigoted humor, however, in which the bigotry is the entire pivot of the joke, is intrinsically harmful, since without the bigotry—that is, without the content predicated on harming some person or class of persons—there would be no joke remaining.

In what follows, I explore several of the ways the types of risks classically associated with sex are expressed in nonsexual social interaction. I discuss the magnified risks of day-to-day social experience that exist for specific classes of people; in particular, I focus on those risks experienced by disabled people and use crip theory as a framework for thinking about social risk. I then discuss risks that may fairly be considered universal—that is, risks that people of any identity might experience as part of their day-to-day social experience.

Ultimately, I show that the sort of attitude we have toward sexual risk—that classes we judge to incur excessive sexual risks should not engage in sex—has implications well beyond sexuality. Such an attitude toward risk leads us to view any given form of social interaction as dispensable for the sake of safety, which, in turn, provides a conveniently benevolent excuse to exclude multiple classes of people from broad swathes of social life.

Embracing and Navigating Social Risk: Resources from Crip Theory

Sex, though risky, is not uniquely risky; rather, it, like other common forms of social interaction, engenders risks and benefits that cannot easily be disentangled from one another. It is, however, the case with conservative ethical discourse that where sex—especially sex that falls under the descriptive rubric of sexual diversity—is concerned, our risk *perception* is heightened while our risk *tolerance* is significantly lowered. What I have attempted to do with the food analogy I made in the previous chapter is to somewhat equalize our risk perception regarding nonsexual interactions. A more thorough theoretical framework, however, is necessary to further equalize our risk perception regarding nonsexual social activities as well as increasing our risk tolerance regarding sexual interaction. Such a framework ought also to put our relationship with social risk into a context that gives it moral direction.

Here, once again, I turn to the thought and experiences of disability studies and activism. In the previous chapter, I used disability studies, and specifically the neurodiversity paradigm, to argue for the moral value of diverse ways of being in the world, especially what I called "perceptual variation," that is, diverse ways of interpreting and responding to sensory input, a category that covers both neuroatypicality and sexual diversity. Here, I turn to crip theory, a movement located at the intersection of disability studies and queer studies that understands "cripness"—like queerness, a reclaimed and reforged slur—to be an expansive, fluid, shifting category and that forges through its intellectual work what Alison Kafer calls a "contestatory" politics. A central thrust of this contestatory politics, following queer theory's interrogation of and resistance to compulsory heterosexuality, is crip theory's resistance to what Robert McRuer calls "compulsory able-bodiedness."

Crip theory is a deeply fruitful theoretical framework here for several reasons. First, crip theory as a field has, through its extensive use of and reference to queer theory, already made the connections between queer and crip experiences, and between normative discourses on the right ways to be sexual and the right ways to be embodied. McRuer thus links compulsory heterosexuality and compulsory able-bodiedness, arguing that these systems are, in fact, interdependent: "The system of compulsory able-bodiedness, which in a sense produces disability, is thoroughly interwoven with the system of compulsory heterosexuality that produces queerness: [in] fact, compulsory heterosexuality is contingent on compulsory able-bodiedness, and vice versa."[9] Indeed, McRuer notes, cripness and queerness are both defined as aberrations from a fixed norm: "The parallel structure of the definitions of ability and sexuality is quite striking: first, to be able-bodied is to be 'free from physical disability,' just as to be heterosexual is to be 'the opposite of homosexual.'"[10] And yet, like queerness, cripness resists the taxonomic fixity of systems of compulsory heterosexuality and able-bodiedness. Rather, it is mutable: as Carrie Sandhal argues, "The term *cripple*, like *queer*, is fluid and ever-changing, claimed by those it did not originally define. . . . The fluidity of both terms makes it likely that their boundaries will dissolve."[11]

Second, and most critically, disabled people often lack the luxury of ignoring risks, both physical and socioemotional, within daily interaction that able-bodied people may take for granted. Depending on the specifics of one's disability, a situation that may be merely inconvenient for or even escape the notice of an abled person may prove life-threatening for a disabled person—for example, the absence of bendable plastic straws from a restaurant or cafeteria might mean that someone cannot drink in that place without risking a potentially fatal choking incident.

Furthermore, crip experience often handily demonstrates the extent to which social-emotional and physical risks are blurred. I have already discussed neurodivergence in the previous chapter; here, interpreting neurodivergence as disability highlights the potential booby traps with which social and emotional interactions may be laden. Inasmuch as neurodivergences such as autism and ADHD render unspoken-yet-foundational social cues and rules difficult to navigate, neurotypical social spaces (which is to say, normative social spaces) are deeply risk laden. And, in addition to the socioemotional pain that can result from botched navigations—a real and significant risk in and of itself—failing to navigate the neurotypical social world according to its normative rules can have inescapably physical consequences: some research on police brutality, for example, suggests that a significant percentage of the victims of fatal police violence (numbers range between 25 and 42 percent) are disabled.[12]

Even when the risks of daily interaction are less immediate than being summarily executed by the state because one's divergent embodiment, perception, or communication render one other (and, it should be noted, there is an enormous overlap here with race and class), disabled people navigate myriad social hazards, ranging from ridicule and social ostracism to lack of accessible toilet facilities to institutionalization and the abuse and neglect that regularly occur in institutions (often in the guise of "therapy" or "treatment"). Harriet McBryde Johnson calls institutions "the disability gulag" and notes that, particularly for those whose disabilities mean they require hourly assistance, remaining free of the gulag depends a great deal on money: "My family could afford hired help [but] I knew my family wasn't like F.D.R.'s or Helen Keller's; they didn't have the means to set me up for life. . . . Whenever my parents scrambled to pay for something unexpected, a part of me saw my freedom hanging in the balance."[13]

Having an obvious and unignorable need for assistance or having obviously divergent access needs can, even if one is free of McBryde Johnson's gulag, carry myriad other risks. The writer and activist Mia Mingus uses the term "forced intimacy" to describe the ways disabled people must render themselves physically, socially, and emotionally vulnerable to meet their basic access needs:

> "Forced Intimacy" is a term I have been using for years to refer to the common, daily experience of disabled people being expected to share personal parts of ourselves to survive in an ableist world. This often takes the form of being expected to share (very) personal information with able bodied people to get basic access, but it also includes forced physical intimacy, especially for those of us who need physical help that often requires touching of our bodies. Forced intimacy can also include the ways that disabled people have to build and sustain emotional intimacy and relationships with someone in order to get access—to get safe, appropriate and good access.[14]

Even if one is able to make their differences and needs less obvious, there are still costs, and disabled people must balance which risks they are willing to bear for the sake of which benefits in intricate and often painful ways. Many autistic writers recount learning to hide stimming behaviors—calming ways of sensory stimulation, like rocking, flapping hands, or chewing on something—and compensate for perceptual and communicative divergences so that they can pass for "normal" or at least merely "weird."

Alyssa Zisk, in an essay in the volume *Loud Hands: Autistic People, Speaking*, notes that passing for merely "weird" meant avoiding McBryde Johnson's gulag (in the form of self-contained special ed classes: "If you're just weird, you can take whatever classes you want"). So Zisk developed coping

strategies, like masking gaze avoidance: "No one notices you're not looking them in the eye if you look at their foreheads."[15] But even being merely
"weird" has social risks, as Julia Bascom notes in an essay in the same volume:
"I was the smartest kid in class. I also did a lot of hiding under my desk, and
I talked funny and moved stiffly, so the other kids formed a club. It had only
one rule, the golden rule: you couldn't talk to Julia."[16] And there are enormous internal, psychological risks to shaping oneself toward the impossible
standard of compulsory abledness. Bascom writes: "I don't need someone
yelling at me to sit down, shut up, stop flapping—I do these things automatically now. No one needs to tell me that I'm worthless—I get that. Message
received, message believed, message drilled into my bones."[17]

It's important to note that I am in no way valorizing the suffering that is
imposed on disabled people by a narrative of compulsory abledness. Such
treatment is, without question, wrong, and any ethical framework worthy of
its name will work toward ending it. Rather, I am noting that disabled people,
of necessity, for the sake of their survival on myriad levels, do not have the
option of ignoring the risks that are inherent in *all* social interactions, in significant part because narratives of compulsory abledness have, for disabled
people, heightened those risks out of all proportion. A theory, therefore, that
is grounded in crip experience is one that must be attentive to risks that compulsory abledness affords nondisabled people the luxury of ignoring. For all
people, nondisabled people included, always face a suite of risks, be they somatic, social, psychological, or even metaphysical, that are part and parcel of
navigating the world. Compulsory abledness serves to rhetorically distance
nondisabled people from those risks, which renders it even more jarring and
offensive when they do encounter them. But that insulation is a fiction.

Indeed, we might say that narratives of compulsory abledness heighten
disabled people's daily social risks to insulate abled people from having to
acknowledge and account for their fair share of risk. And this is another point
of congruence with queerness. For the two points I have made above—that
crip experience regularly encounters and has many nuanced accounts of
risk and that cripness and queerness intersect and are produced by interwoven systems of compulsory being—are themselves connected. For part
(and, as McRuer, reading Judith Butler's *Gender Trouble* onto both queer
and crip experience, notes, an impossible part) of both able-bodied and heterosexual normativity is bodily and social wholeness—understood here not

as a dynamic flourishing (as virtue theorists might put it) but as a static signifier:[18]

> Able-bodied identity, [like heterosexual identity], emerges from disparate features that are supposed to be organized into a seamless and univocal whole: a standard (and "working") number of limbs and digits that are used in appropriate ways (i.e., feet are not used for eating or performing other tasks besides walking; hands are not used as the primary vehicle for language); eyes that see and ears that hear (both consistently and "accurately"); proper dimensions of height and weight (generally determined according to Euro-American standards of beauty); genitalia and other bodily features that are deemed gender-appropriate (i.e., aligned with one of only two possible sexes and in such a way that sex and gender correspond); an HIV-negative serostatus; high energy and freedom from chronic conditions that might in fact impact energy, mobility, and the potential to be awake and "functional" for a standard number of hours each day; freedom from illness or infection (*ideally freedom from the* likelihood *of either illness or infection, particularly HIV infection or sexually transmitted diseases*); acceptable and measurable mental functioning; behaviors that are not disruptive, unfocused, or "addictive"; thoughts that are not unusual or disturbing.[19]

I want to focus in particular on the idea that proper able-bodied heterosexuality is predicated, ideally, not only on *happening* to be free of illness or infection but on being free of the likelihood—that is to say, the risk—of illness or infection. To be straight and abled, ideally, is not just to be free of illness, infection, or impairment in a given moment but to have successfully indemnified oneself against the possibility that one will sustain any kind of lasting damage. And, to strengthen the boundaries of these categories, systems of compulsory heterosexuality and abledness, even as they insist that membership in these categories is the only correct way of being, nevertheless must exclude anyone for whom risk avoidance is obviously impossible. Not incidentally, one technology of this exclusion is to restrict anyone whose identity makes them more unignorably vulnerable from activities these systems have deemed unacceptably risky. The more risk one *must* obviously undertake, in other words, the less risk one should be *allowed* to undertake.

By contrast to this static, composed, and unattainable ideal, McRuer argues, queerness and disability "[refer] to the open mesh of possibilities, gaps, overlaps, dissonances and resonances, lapses and excesses of meaning when the constituent elements of bodily, mental, or behavioral functioning aren't made (or *can't* be made) to signify monolithically."[20] If the absence of risk means that one's being and one's future signifies a single thing, the presence of risk means that there are questions about what one's being and one's future signifies. It means that one is not self-contained, that one lives with uncertainty and multiplicity, and that one's existence is therefore, in some way, disorienting. To be vulnerable to risk, in short, is to contain and live with uncertainty, to not be fully interpretable. It is to require a continued connection and vulnerability, to be open to a continued unfolding and fluidity of meaning. It is to be strange, to be problematic, to be challenging, to be deviant or even freakish. And because risk is deviant, risk is crip and queer.

Highlighting the queerness and cripness of risk in a positive sense is also important, because, even as crip experience demonstrates a heightened level of everyday social risk, it also demonstrates the rich personal and social benefits of practicing a self-aware discipline of thinking about risk and embracing vulnerability. Mingus has coined the term "access intimacy"—as opposed to "forced intimacy," discussed above—to describe the sometimes elusive ease a disabled person experiences when their access needs are met without having to exhaustively explain or justify their needs or even their existence: "Access intimacy is that elusive, hard to describe feeling when someone else 'gets' your access needs. The kind of eerie comfort that your disabled self feels with someone on a purely access level. Sometimes it can happen with complete strangers, disabled or not, or sometimes it can be built over years. It could also be the way your body relaxes and opens up with someone when all your access needs are being met."[21] Access intimacy, for Mingus, also encompasses the sense of affinity necessary for sustainable community formation. It refers, in this sense, to the intimacy that comes both from shared identity and shared understanding:

> Access intimacy is also the intimacy I feel with many other disabled and sick people who have an automatic understanding of access needs out of our shared similar lived experience of the many different ways ableism manifests in our lives. Together, we share a kind of access intimacy that is ground-level, with no need for explanations. Instantly, we can hold the weight, emotion, logistics, isolation, trauma, fear, anxiety and pain of access. I don't have to justify and we are able to start from a place of steel vulnerability. It doesn't mean that our access looks the same, or that we even know what each other's access needs are.[22]

This account therefore adds a critical dimension to our understanding of community and risk. For it highlights that both categories have a great deal to do with communication and, to return to McRuer's thesis, with interpretation. Access intimacy and forced intimacy are, at one level, acts of interpretation, but only one is reciprocal. Forced intimacy expects the disabled person to be a text open to unilateral interpretation, to be simply acted upon. This text has no say in how it offers up its content, in what is divulged from it, how it is handled. It is meant, to use McRuer's language, to signify statically, as is the ideal of compulsory able-bodiedness; even though the disabled body cannot necessarily achieve that abled ideal, it must still *mean* in the same way and be interpreted according to the same hermeneutic as that ideal. Access intimacy, by contrast, describes a fluid and responsive process of mutual interpretation. It is not instant recognition, nor is it an absence of interpretive work. There is still a diversity of meaning and a diversity of interpretive methods; it is, in Bakhtinian terms, heteroglossic. But it removes, as Mingus notes, the need to "justify." It takes for granted that interpretation, if it is not to be an act of violence, must begin with mutuality, with consensual exchange.

Mingus's categories of forced intimacy and access intimacy—both forms of connection and vulnerability, both having to do with access to what one needs to interact with others in private and public space—thus highlight the importance of context for interpreting an action, entity, or state of being. For despite their formal similarities, in lived practice, as Mingus articulates, forced intimacy and access intimacy are very different things. In the first case, vulnerability is exhausting, invasive, threatening, impersonal, and dehumanizing; in the second case, vulnerability is personal, dynamic, affirming, and refreshing. Such is also true, more broadly, of the vulnerability inherent in enfleshedness in general; as Kafer notes, "The blurring of boundaries, the permeability of bodies, the porousness of skin—all take on different meanings depending on whether they are viewed through the prism of institutionalization or as part of a strategy of feminist analysis."[23] Understanding the difference context makes is critical, for even as crip vulnerability is heightened in ways that demonstrate pervasive and systemic ableism, crip agency and practices of radical vulnerability serve as moral discipline and moral witness.

Finally, the importance, here, of crip accounts of risk reminds us once more of the moral value of diverse ways of being, perceiving, and acting, both in and of themselves and within communities. As with the particular case of neurodivergence, disability more broadly generates important models for moral being and action in the world. As Wendell argues, "Like living with cerebral palsy or blindness, living with pain, fatigue, nausea, unpredictable abilities, and/or the imminent threat of death creates different *ways of being* that give valuable perspectives on life and the world."[24] Kafer, commenting on Wendell, elucidates: "Adults who require assistance in the activities of daily life, such as eating, bathing, toileting, and dressing, have opportunities to think through cultural ideals of independence and self-sufficiency; these experiences can potentially lead to productive insights about intimacy, relationship, and interdependence."[25] Crip theory and crip experience offer a diversity of models of moral thought and action for how to recognize risk where we might be tempted to obfuscate it, how to live with that risk, and how to survive and how to flourish in a risk-laden world. Those of us who do not "claim crip" would do well nevertheless to take heed.

Contextualizing Risks in Daily Practice

Discourse about the social-emotional risks of sex tends to go something like this: sexual interaction means exposing yourself intimately and making yourself deeply vulnerable to another person. It can be very painful and psychologically destructive to be so intimate with someone and then be rejected by them; what's more, now the other person has access to a private and intimate part of you that they might use, intentionally or not, to harm you socially. You should, therefore, only engage in sexual interaction with people you know very well and trust without reservation and ideally only with someone to whom you've already made a long-term commitment so that there is no risk of rejection.

The descriptive elements of this discourse are more or less true: sex is, indeed, emotionally and socially risky for the reasons listed above. The salient question, however, is whether it is the *only* form of social intercourse that is risky in these ways. If it is not, as I argue, the only such form, we need to ask whether these risks should impel us to limit similarly risky forms of interaction in the ways described above. And, if not, does it really make sense to limit only sex in those ways?

Sex, to be sure, has characteristics and carries risks and rewards that are particular to it. Most notable among these risks is that of pregnancy, although

it should be noted that not all kinds of sex risk pregnancy and that with current reproductive technologies, it is not necessary to have sex to become
pregnant. (Fortunately, unintended pregnancy due to accidental artificial
insemination seems thus far limited to the script of the TV comedy *Jane the
Virgin*.) And, indeed, pregnancy itself offers an example of a risky chosen
project—as the philosopher Amy Mullin puts it—that societies nevertheless
tend to consider worthwhile in spite of its risks.[26] It is true that societies tend
to consider pregnancy praiseworthy only for certain people—in the contemporary West, this almost always means white, apparently heterosexual,
middle- or upper-class married cisgender women between the approximate
ages of twenty-five and thirty-five. But just because a given pregnancy might
be wanted and planned for by such a person does not mean that it ceases to
be a risky project—although it is true that being white and middle- or upper-
class is, appallingly, correlated with being much less likely to die during pregnancy and childbirth. But monogamous marriage, for example, has no direct
relationship to the risk of hyperemesis gravidarum, preeclampsia, placenta
accreta, or having a baby that is too big to fit through one's pelvis, nor does it
prevent postpartum depression (to name just a few risks). So, at least tacitly,
we recognize that it is morally acceptable and even praiseworthy to accept
certain sexual risks in the name of a chosen project, although it is equally
important to note the extent to which pregnant people, even and perhaps
especially those whose pregnancies society encourages, are infantilized and
denied the dignity of chosen risk.[27]

Yet overall, those risks that are particular to sex are nevertheless connected to the particular characteristics, risks, and rewards of other forms of
social intercourse. Even more important, sex exists with other forms of social
interaction within a continuous, dynamic system of desire and control. One
does not snap into some other moral framework when one enters a sexual
situation; the way one has been conditioned to respond to desire in the presence of others will function in a sexual context as well as in a nonsexual social
context. Indeed, responses to desire that have been made habitual may well
apply even *more* strongly in sexual situations, both because of the instinctual
character of desire and because sexuality is often an integral part of the scaffolding upon which broader social conventions are built.

Sexual interactions—partnered sexual interactions, at least—necessarily
involve negotiating among one's own desires and well-being, the desires and

well-being of at least one other person, relationships with and responsibilities to other persons not present in the encounter, and broader social conventions. This is also the case with other kinds of social interaction. If I am sharing a meal with a friend, I must balance my desire to eat the entire contents of the dish with her desire to eat at least some of it (and perhaps her desire to eat all of it as well). I must balance my desire to order more expensive menu items with my financial health. And I must balance my desire to lick the plate with the knowledge that it is broadly considered rude to do so in public.

Sexual interactions carry with them risks of illness or injury—both physical and emotional. As the entire focus of this book should indicate, STIs are a serious public health issue. BDSM practices and even vanilla sexual encounters that become exuberant or careless risk physical injury. And the intimacy, emotional significance, and vulnerability inherent in a sexual encounter entail considerable risk of psychological and emotional pain. These risks also occur, however, with other types of social interaction. To take the example of sharing meals again: eating carries risks of contracting food poisoning or parasites, and preparing food carries risks of cuts and burns. It may be tempting to argue that these physical risks are of a different type altogether—surely a bout of food poisoning or a cut from a kitchen knife is nothing compared to syphilis or HIV! But statistics beg to differ: the Centers for Disease Control estimates that there are 179 million cases of foodborne illness annually in the United States, resulting in 486,777 annual hospitalizations and 6,189 deaths.[28] The US Fire Administration reports that cooking was the cause of 50.3 percent of all 364,300 estimated residential building fires—including an estimated 118 fatal ones—and 29.9 percent of all 96,800 nonresidential building fires in 2016.[29]

The social aspects of sharing meals also carry emotional risks: food is invested with all sorts of social and personal significance, and articulating gustatory needs and desires can be quite fraught. Both preparers and consumers of shared meals may experience significant—and reasonable—anxiety about exposure to physical dangers, pleasing others, and following social conventions. The social-emotional risks of cooking and eating also interact with and magnify the physical risks. Imagine you are a guest at a dinner party in which you are unsure whether some of the dishes are entirely safe to eat. All other things being equal, you would probably avoid the questionable dishes. But if the host has clearly put a great deal of effort and emotional investment into the meal, perhaps you might eat some of the questionable dishes anyway, for the sake of sparing the host's feelings. Or imagine that you are cooking while entertaining friends in the kitchen; you may be sharing wine or beer at the time. Perhaps, because of your divided attention or the alcohol or both, you are less attentive to matters of knife and fire safety than you would otherwise be.

Yet it is precisely navigating these physical and social risks that makes social eating such an important school for wise personal and social conduct. Eating would not shape us as moral and social actors as it does if it were without risk, because without risk we do not change and so we do not learn. And when the preparation and sharing of meals go right, I find that little compares to the sense of intimacy, care, and connection that can occur around the dinner table. In addition to being valuable in their own right, the shared sensory pleasures of a well-prepared meal can, if navigated well, be conducive to a multitude of social goods and can help foster the sorts of social relationships—caring, supportive, and intellectually generative romantic partnerships, friendships, mentorships, and so forth—that build good, dynamic, and diverse communities. And I think that few mainstream voices would contradict me if I said that this suite of sensory, psychological, and social goods were well worth the risks of cooking and eating, both in and of itself and as a social activity. (Though it is worth noting that one way dominant power structures marginalize those they consider deviant is to restrict their ability to safely eat in public—consider the recent popularity of public bans on plastic straws, which allow many disabled people to drink safely, or the woman who, in the spring of 2018, called the police on a Black family barbecuing in an Oakland, California, park because she considered them "disruptive.")

When we think about the activities through which we experience social pleasure, build social relationships, and learn about respectful and ethical interpersonal conduct, we don't tend to think of them primarily as risk activities, even though, again, we wouldn't learn from them if they were not. And we must, I suspect, put ourselves through far more contortions about just who counts as a moral agent to argue that some classes must be excluded from these activities, which we cast as universals. But even something as "tame" and basic as eating carries similar risks, on many levels, as sex does. And, like eating, sex shapes us as moral and social actors in fundamental and ongoing ways.

Risk, therefore, is a poor criterion, at least on its own, through which to restrict some classes of people from engaging in fundamental activities of moral development and social exchange, sex included. It is an equally poor criterion for restricting some ways of engaging in those activities over and against others. It is, however, a deeply fruitful category through which to understand the ways in which those activities shape us as actors. And because of its basic queerness (in the term's most fundamental sense, that of being strange, unsettling, discomfiting), it invites us to consider who has been excluded from "proper" expressions of those activities and why. Risk is not something to be romanticized. It often points to the possibility of real harm. But it cannot ever be avoided fully, and it is therefore something to be engaged with and learned from. For, indeed, there can be no learning—moral learning very much included—without it.

Livability and Discernment: Concepts for an Ethic of Social Risk

Sexual actors, and social actors more generally, thus must constantly weigh a matrix of risks, desires, and actual and potential goods when deciding which interactions they shall engage in. When we engage in this process of moral weighing, we are trying to find patterns of sexual and social interaction that are livable. A situation is livable when a balance is achieved between one's needs and desires (including those needs and desires that arise from pre-cognitive instincts or urges), the needs and desires of individual others with whom one interacts, and the basic structures of the social orders in which one lives, such that flourishing is accessible to everyone and that no one experiences unbearable hardship. By flourishing, I do not mean in the sense of the term as used, for example, in the field of positive psychology, that is, "within an optimal range of human functioning, one that connotes goodness, generativity, growth, and resilience."[30] Such a definition seems to me to at least partially beg the question ("goodness" as a component of "optimal functioning," for example, is "indexed by happiness, satisfaction, and superior functioning"), and terms like "optimal functioning" tend to slouch quickly toward outright ableism.[31] Rather, by flourishing, I mean the more subjective ability to carry out and take reasonable pleasure—of which one is the ultimate arbiter—in one's activities of daily living, social relationships, and chosen projects. By unbearable hardship, I mean burdens that cause enough physical or psychological hardship to substantially interfere with one's flourishing or burdens that cause one to feel a significant and painful disjunction between one's understanding of who one is (identity, values, beliefs, and so on) and the roles one is expected to carry out in one's social context.

Livability is not a universally trumping value. Research into pedophilia, for example, seems to indicate that it functions very much like a sexual orientation, such that denying sexual access to children may well be "unlivable" in this sense for at least some exclusive pedophiles. Yet clearly, to allow pedophiles sexual access to children would be unlivable for those children and would constitute a dereliction of social and individual duties to protect those who are unable or less able to protect themselves. Thus, there are cases in which what is "livable" for a particular individual or community is so deeply at odds with the basic needs of other individuals or of a broader community, because it would inflict clear and overwhelming harm on others, that it cannot be permitted by a moral society.

In many cases, though, finding a livable balance does not entail such a clear and one-sided weighing of harms, risks, and benefits; rather, it involves a complex balancing of these among multiple interests. Such balancing is not always easy, and livability emphatically does not exclude hardship, self-discipline, extended and intense efforts, or potentially painful choices. Rather, it is a question of distinguishing between manageable, workable hardship versus hardship that begins to take over one's life and drown out everything else.

Livability as a concept also gives more clarity to the idea of *sexual fulfillment*, since it offers a robust and specific way of speaking of sexual fulfillment—and in particular of the diversity of sexual preferences and urges that people experience and that, in most cases, they would do well to have the opportunity to explore—that does not fall into the trap of claiming that a given pattern of desire or action is "natural" or not. This trap has been difficult to avoid for some contemporary writers (especially those connected to the field of evolutionary psychology) who ask, for example, whether monogamy is "natural."[32] But "naturalness," so deployed, is not a helpful or meaningful moral category.[33] Any number of behaviors that are unambiguously morally problematic—xenophobia, violent aggression, domination of weaker individuals or groups—are also quite "natural," insofar as they reliably occur to some extent in nearly every known cultural and social configuration. As Dewey puts it, "Nature has no preference for good things over bad things; its mills turn out any kind of grist indifferently."[34] It is not therefore obvious that the use of cultural tools to regulate "natural" (in the sense of "instinctive" or "given") urges and behaviors is in and of itself harmful. To argue against a given sociosexual convention on the grounds that it suppresses natural instincts or desires does not by itself tell us whether it is harmful to suppress that instinct or desire.

Nevertheless, when these writers ask whether a given sociosexual convention is natural, they *do* identify an important aspect of sexuality. Desires and instincts *do* have major components that are "given"—that is, by the time we are aware of them, they are more or less in place, regardless of their ultimate etiology—and durable, and changing or suppressing those components may be difficult or impossible. When we ask whether monogamy, for example, is natural, what we may mean is whether it is practically workable or desirable to insist that someone who is strongly and durably inclined toward nonmonogamy (for whatever reason) nevertheless adopt a monogamous lifestyle. Livability as a concept accounts for this durability of desire as a valid moral datum in and of itself, *without* resorting to dubious claims of naturalness.

To assess what is livable for oneself, one's immediate fellows, and one's community and to balance potentially conflicting risks and goods require cultivating the virtue of discernment. Discernment, by which I mean the capacity to observe, analyze, weigh, and make careful judgments concerning information related to risks and goods as they may affect oneself and others, is a key virtue for the ongoing practice of risk management. Importantly, discernment is not synonymous with expertise, at least in any specific sense: any moral agent can cultivate and practice discernment regardless of whether they have become expert in any given field or profession. Discernment requires seeking out relevant information and attempting to understand and sift it fairly, from multiple perspectives; this can also mean recognizing where one is *not* expert and, where necessary, seeking expert assistance.

Along these lines, discernment also requires admitting the limits of one's knowledge and understanding and seeking help where necessary, feasible, and safe. Further, it requires understanding that everyone will have gaps in their knowledge and capacity for understanding and that these will vary among persons and communities depending on a variety of factors and that, conversely, so too will particular strengths in understanding. This, along with the recognition that each person is the ultimate judge of what is livable for them, means that part of discernment is also practicing charity regarding any assumptions one might make concerning whether another agent is in fact practicing this virtue. I might, for example, be tempted to judge someone who enjoys free-climbing rocks to be exercising insufficient discernment concerning risks to their physical safety. But, if I myself am to be discerning about my judgment, I must admit that (1) I am quite afraid of heights, which is going to condition my immediate response, and (2) I am unlikely to have access to the details of the climber's life such that I could even begin to judge what is livable for them. Perhaps free-climbing rocks is one of the only forms of physical activity they actually enjoy (as the equally risky equestrianism is for me). Perhaps it helps them manage a mental illness. Perhaps they just enjoy it enough that it is, for them, a core part of livability.

It's tempting to assume that someone who regularly engages in obviously risky behaviors, including and perhaps especially, risky sexual behaviors, must lack discernment. This is all the more true when the behaviors have a clear link to bodily appetites, which we're used to thinking about as anarchic and unreasonable. And it's even more the case when someone who regularly engages in risky behaviors doesn't appear to take what one might think of as obvious risk-mitigation measures. It seems clear, for example, that someone who has multiple sexual partners and doesn't regularly get tested for STIs is exercising an egregious lack of discernment. But in fact, that description doesn't give anyone sufficient information to make that judgment call. Perhaps that person doesn't have reliable access to an STI clinic, whether for reasons of cost, transportation, or something else. Perhaps they have experienced violence, coercion, or some other maltreatment at the hands of medical providers, and clinics are not, in their experience, safe places. Perhaps one of their partners is abusive and would become violent if they encountered evidence of STI treatment. Perhaps there is some contingency that is beyond my ability to imagine. In such a case, it may be that the person in question, far from lacking discernment, is demonstrating a supererogatory level of discernment, weighing threats to livability and indeed life and livelihood with a level of skill that should, in fact, impress any observer.[35]

Importantly, recognizing this doesn't change the fact that we all have obligations to protect our own well-being and that of others. Awareness and communication of one's STI status is a moral duty for any sexually active person. But being discerning about the limits of one's own ability to judge others' virtues and vices reminds us that all too often we live within structures that simultaneously make it impossible to carry out our duties to one another and then blame us for failing to overcome the structures' impossible hurdles. In such a world, exercising discernment in a way that enables individual and collective livability as well as one can is not just excusable; it is exemplary. As Sharon Welch puts it in her account of a feminist ethic of risk, "Actions begin with the recognition that far too much has been lost and there are no clear means of restitution. The fundamental risk constitutive of this ethic is the decision to care and to act although there are no guarantees of success."[36]

An astute reader might, at this point, raise the criticism that my discussion here of risk and pleasure and my emphasis on discernment and on risk takers, especially sexual risk takers, as *rational* agents, is perhaps insufficiently attentive to the *irrational* characteristics of sex, sexuality, and desire in general—to, as a reader of an earlier draft of this manuscript put it, "the gaps between the virtues we would all ideally exercise and the reality of our failure to exercise these virtues consistently because of how humans are." This critique is an important one, and it's especially relevant to any discussion of risk—not least because the gap between what we'd ideally do and what we're *likely* to do is yet another risk we must navigate, in sexual encounters as well as in social encounters more broadly! In fact, the next two chapters, as well as the conclusion, explore various facets of the risks engendered by this gap.

Nevertheless, there is a reason why I've focused on the ways in which sexual decision-making can be and indeed is rational. This is not because I think we are all Mr. Data in bed (obviously we are not) or because I think the traditionally rational faculties are better or more worthy of study. Rather, it is because so much writing on sexuality and sexual encounters, especially within our field, egregiously overemphasizes the irrational, uncontrolled, and even animalistic qualities of sexuality, treating sexual urges as forces of nature that overwhelm any rational decision-making and treating sexual "deviants" as out of moral control. It's also important to point out that the boundaries between rational and irrational decisions and actions are far fuzzier and more fluid than regnant accounts treat them as being—and that where those accounts draw lines between rational and irrational is heavily conditioned by and reproductive of the power hierarchies in which they are invested.[37]

In this chapter and the preceding one, I laid out some reasons why the ways we carry out those bodily appetites we're used to thinking of as anarchic and unreasonable involve far more reason and far less unruliness than we might think. These behaviors are inextricably linked to and conditioned by complex social structures and processes of decision-making, they help develop a range of different perspectives and virtues that are valuable to both individuals and communities, and they help build a life that supports flourishing. Even so, however, it can be difficult to internalize these observations, and so the temptation to assume a lack of discernment in others remains. Being discerning about our own judgment and cultivating humility about the information we do and do not have access to are important antidotes to this temptation. And, in doing so, perhaps we can cultivate the discipline necessary to think more carefully, more humanely, and more livably about sexual risk and social risk more broadly.

Transition: Risk and the Rabbis

Where might we find constructive treatments of social risk in classical Jewish sources? In chapter 4, I argue that the Mishnah's account of ritual impurity, especially as demonstrated in tractate Zavim, offers a portrait of engagement with ubiquitous social contagion and the ever-present risk of contracting it, that has much to recommend to it as a way of thinking through contemporary management of STIs. In chapter 5, I argue that the rabbinic bet midrash, as we encounter it in classical rabbinic literature, is what I call a risk-conditioned community: that is, it is a community whose central, uniting affinity is an acknowledged risk activity and in which the techniques of self-formation it encourages are significantly shaped by the need to competently manage that risk. There, I use the well-known Oven of Akhnai text (B. Bava Metsia 59a–b), which depicts the entire sagely assembly engaging in a case of interpretive edge play, to explore the ways in which risk is central to the bet midrash as a whole.

Here, as a transition between what I have done thus far and the case studies I will discuss in the next two chapters, I want to briefly engage a rabbinic story that touches on the importance of risk for individual actors. The story of Rabbi Yoḥanan and Resh Lakish in Bavli Bava Metsia 84a has been much analyzed by scholars of sex, gender, and rabbinic text, notably R. R. Neis and Daniel Boyarin, for its deployment of what Neis calls "visual eros" and its homoerotic themes.[38] Directly preceding this passage, for example, we are told that the androgynous and famously beautiful Rabbi Yoḥanan has a habit of loitering outside the mikveh.[39] In this way, he hopes that the women leaving it—newly in a state of ritual purity and likely going home to have sex with their husbands—will, according to the prevailing contemporary belief that what one saw around the time of a child's conception affected their physical characteristics, conceive children just as beautiful as he is. Additionally, the story plays consciously on R. Yoḥanan's androgyny and the emotional and possibly sexual intensity of his relationship with Resh Laḳish; in its form, it reads neatly and hauntingly as a romantic tragedy.

In addition to these themes, however, this passage may also be read as a poignant and devastating meditation on the risks of life-giving social relations—and on the costs of eliminating those risks. The perils of Torah study as an activity and of interpersonal relationships and intense emotional vulnerability, as well as the crushing damage of their absence in the life of one who needs them, are all present and on clear display. In this way, the story itself presents a way into the ways risks both great and small are subjects of complex moral significance within classical rabbinic texts.

In this text, the bandit Resh Laḳish encounters the beautiful Rabbi Yoḥanan bathing on the banks of the Jordan River; mistaking him for a woman, he vaults across the river on his javelin—which is definitely *not* symbolic of anything—presumably intending to take "her" by force. Rabbi Yoḥanan, however, responds to the threat of an armed bandit accosting him with his own preferred weapons, those of words and wit. Once Resh Laḳish realizes his error, he attempts to engage, commenting on Rabbi Yoḥanan's beauty and androgyny, but he is quickly bested. Rabbi Yoḥanan offers Resh Laḳish his sister's hand in marriage, as well as his teaching. When Resh Laḳish accepts, he then discovers the trade-off, the unspoken risk: having taken up the weapons of the mind and tongue, he no longer has the great physical strength he only just displayed:

> One day Rabbi Yoḥanan was bathing in the Jordan. Resh Laḳish saw him and, thinking he was a woman, stuck his lance into the Jordan and vaulted to the other side after him.
>
> [When Rabbi Yoḥanan saw Resh Laḳish,] he said to him, "Your strength for Torah!"
>
> [Resh Laḳish] said to him, "Your beauty for women!"
>
> He said to him, "If you return [away from banditry and toward Torah,] I will give you my sister, who is more beautiful than I am!"

He took it upon himself [to study Torah.]
He wanted to go back to collect his clothes, but he was unable to.
[R. Yoḥanan] taught him Torah and Mishnah, and made him a fellow
great man.[40]

Rabbi Yoḥanan brings Resh Lakish into the rabbinic community first as his
student—he makes him "a great man," a sage who is learned in Torah and
skilled in argumentation—and then as his colleague and study partner, a role
that involves engaging one another in fierce, pitched verbal battles. The two
develop, in other words, an intellectually, emotionally, spiritually socially,
and possibly sexually intense bond—one that's further cemented by ties of
blood, since Resh Lakish has married Rabbi Yoḥanan's sister. In multiple,
deeply meaningful senses, they have become family, with all the vulnerability and mutual dependence that entails.

Then, one day, the bonds rupture:

One day they were disputing [a *baraita*] in the bet midrash: the sword, the
knife, the dagger, the spear, a hand-scythe, a harvest-scythe—from when are
they susceptible to impurity? From the time their manufacture is complete.
    And when is their manufacture complete? R. Yoḥanan said: from when
one forges them in the furnace. Resh Lakish said: from when one polishes
them in water.

It is not accidental that the argument that destroys this relationship—
which started with a javelin and is based on intense and ferocious verbal
sparring—also concerns weaponry. Different physical objects become susceptible to ritual impurity under different conditions; here the parties have
an authoritative tradition that states that blades become susceptible when
their manufacture is complete. The disagreement concerns what counts
as "complete." Rabbi Yoḥanan offers an opinion; Resh Lakish contradicts
him in a way that demonstrates greater knowledge of the process of making
blades. At this point, Rabbi Yoḥanan hits back below the belt:

[R. Yoḥanan] said to him, "A bandit knows his banditry!"
    [Resh Lakish] retorted: "So what benefit have you brought me? There
they call me 'Rabbi,' and here they call me 'Rabbi'!"
    [R. Yoḥanan] retorted: "Did I benefit you?! For I brought you under the
pinions of the Divine Presence!"
    R. Yoḥanan's mind was sickened, and Resh Lakish fell gravely ill.

Resh Laḳish, R. Yoḥanan snaps, knows this technical detail because he's still, at heart, the bandit he was when they met—a claim that humiliates Resh Laḳish in front of his peers and wounds him as much as any blade. He retorts that if that's how Rabbi Yoḥanan is going to treat him, there was no point in all this—after all, he was already a leader and a great man among the bandits! Rabbi Yoḥanan shoots back that Resh Laḳish ought to be grateful, since he brought him back to the divine presence. The whole exchange sickens both of them—Resh Laḳish gravely so.

A relationship such as theirs, based as it is in verbal battle, always risked this. Now the risk has been realized. R. Yoḥanan's sister—who clearly understands the stakes in a way that her brother, at the moment, does not—pleads with him to unbend and apologize, correctly arguing that lives hang in the balance. Yet, as is often the fate of obviously correct women in the Talmud, she goes unheeded:

> [R. Yoḥanan's] sister came weeping [to him]. She said to him: "Act for the sake of my children!"
> He said to her: "Leave your orphaned children, I will keep them alive." [Jer. 49:11]
> She said to him: "Act for the sake of my widowhood!"
> He said to her [the rest of the verse]: "And let your widows trust in me."

Here, Rabbi Yoḥanan is, not to put too fine a point on it, being a smug jackass. Not only is he responding to his sister's life-and-death pleas with clever proof texts; he is specifically and blithely using proof texts that appeal to eschatological divine justice in a situation that is, in fact, well within R. Yoḥanan's power to mend.

Only after it is too late and Resh Laḳish dies does R. Yoḥanan grasp the seriousness of what has occurred: "Resh Laḳish died. R. Yoḥanan pined greatly for him." If the risks of the partnership and its central interpretive activity proved fatal to Resh Laḳish, it is the risks of its loss that finally overwhelm R. Yoḥanan. Seeing him overcome with and impaired by his grief, the sages send him a new study partner—a "replacement goldfish," if you will, like the narrative trope of a parent who replaces their child's deceased pet with a superficially similar one—R. Elazar ben Pedat.[41] But ben Pedat fails to understand that it is precisely the risk, the sharpness, of R. Yoḥanan's partnership with Resh Laḳish that makes it life-sustaining:

The Rabbis said: Who will go and calm him? Let R. Elazar ben Pedat go, for
his statements are sharp.
  [R. Elazar ben Pedat] went and sat before [R. Yoḥanan]. For everything
R. Yoḥanan would say, he would say to him, "There is a baraita that supports
you."
  [R. Yoḥanan] said: Are you like the son of Laḳish!? When I would assert
something, the son of Laḳish would trouble me with twenty-four problems,
and I would answer back at him twenty-four answers, and the tradition
would expand of its own accord! And you say to me, "There is a baraita that
supports you?!" Do I not know that my statements are fabulous?!

The sages' intervention fails, only sharpening R. Yoḥanan's sense of loss. He
becomes insane, only finding relief when the sages pray for his death:

  [R. Yoḥanan] wound about, tearing his clothes, weeping, and saying,
  "Where are you, son of Laḳish? Where are you, son of Laḳish?" He
  screamed until his reason left him.
  The Rabbis prayed for mercy upon him, and so he died.

What is occurring here? First, the relationship between the two rabbis is
obviously a risky one: it eventually claims the life of both rabbis, the force of
whose rhetoric, bolstered by the metaphysical power of the divinely charged
words they are working with, explicitly holds the power to enervate, sicken,
and kill. As if to underscore this point, martial metaphors—the spear, the
dagger—abound, and Resh Laḳish's background as a violent outlaw is consciously juxtaposed with R. Yoḥanan's intellectual pugnaciousness.
  Second, both main protagonists shape one another and are shaped by their
risky partnership. R. Yoḥanan, here, clearly shapes Resh Laḳish, making him
a Torah scholar and a "great man," but the converse occurs, too: Resh Laḳish
has shaped R. Yoḥanan into someone who delights in such an intense intellectual, social, and emotional relationship and comes to require it to survive.
As Jeffrey Rubenstein writes, "For R. Yoḥanan, the lack of intense dialectical
debate was essentially a fate worse than death. He craved heated intellectual
combat, not a yes-man to confirm the veracity of his pronouncements."[42]
Further, the partnership itself is shaped as a social unit, whose contours become clearest in its loss: it is the utter lack of risk in the interchanges with ben
Pedat that renders these stultifying and only highlights how the potential for
defeat and injury in R. Yoḥanan and Resh Laḳish's exchanges was precisely
what made them constructive and life-giving.

We can read the concept of dignity of risk and its relationship to disability as operative here, as well, particularly if we posit that R. Yoḥanan is so overwhelmed by his grief that he becomes impaired by it. R. Yoḥanan's community recognizes that his pain is connected to the loss of his partner, and so they send him a replacement, but why send a yes-man like ben Pedat? Such may not have been their intention, since the sages in fact seem to judge that ben Pedat should prove a worthy replacement, reasoning that "his traditions are sharp," so why doesn't ben Pedat live up to his reputation? Likely he was acting in deference to R. Yoḥanan's seniority, but it is worth considering that he was also moved to treat R. Yoḥanan gently because of his illness. Perhaps, ben Pedat reasoned, someone in such a state as R. Yoḥanan's is in no position to handle the risks of pitched rabbinic debate! R. Yoḥanan thus finds himself with a "safe"—and lifeless!—replacement for the relationship whose loss has disabled him. And the putative "safe" choice turns out to be even more dangerous, for it highlights the enormity of his loss and plunges him into fatal despair.

I don't highlight this story to argue that it presents a good overall model for risk in social ethics—indeed, *everyone* in this story could and should have been far wiser and more humane in their social risk-management practices. I do, however, think it provides one piece of textual support for Jewishly grounding my argument that risk is something that constantly and fundamentally shapes us as moral actors. It also introduces the argument, which I take up in greater detail in chapter 5, that classical rabbinic texts do not just tolerate social risk but that they situate particular kinds of social risk as central organizing affinities for their paradigm community, the rabbinic bet midrash. Finally, this story offers a poignant reminder that risk, even mortal risk, can be, for many, a crucial part of what makes life livable. R. Yoḥanan and Resh Laḳish's relationship was intense, tempestuous, and risky, and for Resh Laḳish it proved ultimately deadly. Yet for R. Yoḥanan, without that relationship, intrinsic to which was real and serious risk, flourishing was impossible, and life was not worth living. We can and should condemn much of his behavior, but when we think about what roles risk plays in our lives, we'd do well to remember his end.

PART II

Case Studies on Community and Risk

In the previous three chapters, I have canvassed an approach to reading and thinking with text and with sexuality that I argue cultivates the broader virtues of empirical justice, hermeneutic competency, wise risk management, and diverse interdependence. In the remaining chapters, I apply this approach to two case studies, bringing selected rabbinic texts into conversation with the management of STIs and organized BDSM practice. In doing so, I show specific ways in which this approach can cultivate the virtues I've mentioned and the practical importance of those virtues in our daily lives as socially engaged creatures.

The following two chapters bring together the claims I have made in the previous section through specific, concrete examples. Chapter 4 uses mishnaic ritual purity discourse to articulate a moral model for understanding and managing STIs. Chapter 5 treats the activity of rabbinic text interpretation, as it is portrayed within rabbinic text itself, as a chosen risk activity that constitutes communities and shapes identities, and uses that as a lens to consider and evaluate the virtues—and vices!—cultivated and demonstrated by organized BDSM communities. In each case, I show how an understanding of sex as social intercourse better accounts for the concrete realities of actual sexual phenomena, and I demonstrate how attending to the social functions of the subject matter of specific rabbinic texts helps them generate more detailed and useful guidance for contemporary ethicists.

Each case study addresses a different aspect or iteration of risk and the relevant virtues of wise risk management and diverse interdependence. My first case study, that of STIs, deals with the risk of contagion, something that is often what one might call a "known unknown." Contagion is a risk that can be substantially known and managed but never completely so. It is a risk that is generally not sought out but almost always eventually encountered—though people may seek out a certain activity with full awareness that they are increasing their risk of contagion—and so I use it to think about the ethics of encountering the kinds of social risks that are ambient, unlooked for, and ever-present. My second case study, of BDSM, deals with the kinds of risks that people consciously and actively court for their own sake. Here, the risk is not a byproduct of a desired activity or experience but the desired activity or experience itself. I use this case study to think about the moral disciplines an individual or a community may cultivate when they actively seek out risk. Both cases also address the variation inherent among risks themselves and the ways actors and communities experience and respond to risks, as well as some of the ways communities can intentionally organize themselves around that variation.

Finally, a note on sources: throughout the next two chapters, I rely heavily on Mira Balberg's *Purity, Body, and Self in Early Rabbinic Literature* and Beth Berkowitz's *Execution and Invention: Death Penalty Discourse in Early Rabbinic and Christian Cultures*, respectively, as the main guides for my readings of the relevant primary texts, perhaps to what appears to be the exclusion of other relevant work in these areas. It is certainly not the case that Balberg and Berkowitz have written the only or final words on the respective topics of ritual purity in the Mishnah and rabbinic execution. Jodi Magness, Stuart Miller, and Yair Furstenberg, for example, have all done pivotal recent work on Second Temple and rabbinic impurity.[1] Berkowitz's study, as she herself notes, builds in important ways on the work of scholars like Moshe Halbertal, Yair Lorberbaum, Devora Steinmetz, and Aharon Shemesh.[2] Other recent scholarly work on violence and ritualized punishment in rabbinic literature includes that of Ishay Rosen-Zvi and Mika Ahuvia.[3]

These chapters, however, are not meant to be comprehensive surveys of the subjects of rabbinic impurity and rabbinic execution. Rather, these chapters treat Balberg and Berkowitz as dialogue partners and theoretical resources, in a similar way to how one might engage at length with more obviously "theoretical" thinkers—just as one might offer, say, a Levinasian or Bakhtinian reading of a given primary text. My goal in these chapters, then, is to explore what each scholar's particular approach can yield in this sort of dialogue.

4. STIs

Infection, Impurity, and Managing Social Contagion

STIS ARE ONE OF the paradigmatic risks of sexual interaction; no doubt many of us remember being shown appallingly magnified slides of genital warts as part of our high school sex ed curricula's attempts to scare and disgust us into abstinence. STIs sit at the intersection of individual sexuality and public concern. Further, because STIs are issues of public concern that are transmissible by specific forms of social and physical contact, they offer a strong parallel to rabbinic frameworks of ritual purity and, in doing so, provide a helpful demonstration of the hermeneutic methodology I proposed in the previous chapter.

When we talk about STIs, there are four critical things to know: First, STIs are incredibly common—and, in fact, far more common than they need to be.[1] Second, STIs are real risks that can have important consequences on both an individual and a public level.[2] Third, those risks are eminently manageable. Fourth and finally, the public perception of STIs, the seriousness of their consequences, and the extent to which the tools available to manage them are used effectively and justly are inextricably entangled with multiple systems of gender, sex, race, class, and ability-based oppression.

STI risk cannot be eliminated, but it can be managed. Simply exhorting people to avoid sexual risk doesn't work: abstinence-only sex education neither prevents people from engaging in premarital sex nor reduces rates of unplanned pregnancy or STI transmission. Effective management strategies do exist, but they are complex and multifactorial.[3] Modern medical science has developed treatments, vaccines, and physical and chemical methods of prophylaxis that make consensual sex, for those who have access to these wonders, safer than it has ever been at any point in human history.

However, STIs are far from a strictly technological problem. Techno-logical advances are an essential component of STI management, but they are not sufficient, because STIs are socially transmitted among fundamen-tally social beings. STIs demonstrate the extent to which social behavior occurs in and tangibly affects the material world. The social components of STI transmission affect the efficacy of our technological tools for STI man-agement in serious ways. Inappropriate antibiotic use and nonchalance about the prevention of bacterial STIs has led to a worrying rise in antibiotic-resis-tant gonorrhea. Inconsistent compliance with antiretroviral drug regimens makes drug-resistant HIV strains a serious concern.[4] Suboptimal rates of vaccination against cancer-causing strains of human papillomavirus (HPV) allow innumerable preventable (and sometimes fatal) cancers to arise. Dis-parities in access to medical care, combined with stigma against people who are infected and faulty reasoning about the moral effect of proactive STI prevention and sex education, mean that potentially effective methods of treatment and prevention fail to reach those who need them most. The best possible medical technologies are useless if not adopted. Social strategies for managing STIs are critical to encourage the widespread adoption of effective modes of treatment and prevention.

STI rates generally (though not always) follow predictable patterns: ra-cial minorities, sexual minorities (with the notable exception of women who exclusively have sex with women), and economically disadvantaged populations tend to bear a higher burden of risk both in terms of infection rates and in terms of access to prevention, testing, and treatment.[5] Further-more, the extent to which we as a society fail to adequately manage STIs is not, primarily, a technological problem. We know we have a range of very successful options for both prevention and treatment, although the rise of antibiotic-resistant bacteria, gonorrhea in particular, is a notable and deeply worrisome exception. Rather, our problems are largely economic and social: communities lack sufficient access to these effective interventions, and, more insidiously, the social climate around matters of sexual health makes frank and accurate discussion of STI prevention and treatment socially and pol-itically difficult and makes it shameful to seek out help or even to know and disclose one's STI status.

Indeed, the dominant discourses surrounding sexually transmitted infections have overwhelmingly been ones of otherness. Even in antiquity, sexually linked maladies seem to have carried some association with people and behaviors outside the bounds of social acceptability.[6] During the Italian outbreak of 1496, which the Italians referred to at the time as the *morbis gallicus*, or "French disease," and which most historians take to be the first recorded outbreak of syphilis, Gilino of Ferrera, who was also one of the first to connect the disease to sex with an infected individual,[7] wrote that "the Supreme Creator, now full of wrath against us for our dreadful sins, punishes us with the cruelest of ills, which has now spread not only through Italy but across the whole of Christendom."[8] Italians also blamed Jews and Arabs who had recently been expelled from Spain in 1492, many of whom had taken refuge in Italy.[9] By 1526, European writers had begun to connect syphilis's origin to Columbus's voyages to the New World, which offered in Native Americans a convenient and mutually agreeable scapegoat.[10]

Otherness encompassed not only race and ethnicity but also class and especially gender. Women—prostitutes in particular—were understood as potential sources of infection and as dangerous to men. In 1497 Gilino of Ferrara and Widman of Tubingen advised men to avoid contact with infected women.[11] By the modern era, syphilis, both in Europe and the US, was strongly linked to marginalized racial and ethnic groups—Jews and colonized peoples in Europe, and, in the US, immigrants and especially African Americans.[12] Progressive Era (1890–1920) responses to venereal disease (VD), as it was then called, focused on eradicating prostitution, painting "loose women" as a threat to public health; this rhetoric of the dangerous woman intensified during the two world wars.[13] HIV/AIDS was famously characterized as the "gay plague" (its original medical name was gay-related immune deficiency), and it continues to conjure strong associations with race, class, addiction, and sexual orientation.

If the origins of STIs lay outside the dominant culture, STIs within that culture were nevertheless understood as a moral check on members' baser impulses. The rapid spread of syphilis throughout Europe in the fifteenth and sixteenth centuries was quickly figured as a manifestation of divine wrath. In 1949, shortly after penicillin was found to effectively treat syphilis, John Stokes, a syphilis expert at the University of Pennsylvania, worried that "if extramarital sexual relations lead neither to significant illness nor unwanted parenthood, only a few intangibles of the spirit remain to guide children of the new era from an outmoded past into an unbridled future."[14] Early in the AIDS epidemic, the Moral Majority executive Ronald S. Godwin criticized federal spending on AIDS research because it was "a commitment to spend our tax dollars on research to allow these diseased homosexuals to go back to their perverted practices without any standards of accountability."[15] Recently, there has been opposition to widespread vaccination of preteens against cancer-causing strains of HPV, partly due to the (demonstrably incorrect) perception that it will encourage youth to initiate sexual activity earlier.[16]

These constructions of STIs seem constant even as the character of public discourse around them has changed. In the United States, for example, Progressive Era reformers and physicians called for frank discussion of VD, arguing that only candid sex education could help stem the infectious tide. They also opposed the double standard of sexual behavior, according to which women were chaste creatures whose virtues lay in their sexual purity while men were libidinous animals who required sex, instead arguing that proper social hygiene, health practices, and moral standards obligated both men and women to preserve their virginities until marriage. Even as these reformers challenged what they saw as dangerous and outdated norms, however, VD remained a threat originating from outside the ranks of good society, especially the lower socioeconomic classes.[17] And if Progressives and social hygienists sought to eliminate the sexual double standard, they nevertheless implored men to control their physical drives while exhorting women—still largely painted as asexual—to demand a higher standard of restraint from men for the sake of their own protection. Further, this leveling only applied to "proper" women. Prostitutes were another matter entirely. As Allan M. Brandt puts it, "An 'innocent' woman could only get venereal disease from a 'sinful' man. But the man could only get venereal disease from a 'fallen woman.'"[18] The common epithet "social disease" even claimed an identity between VD and the "social evil" of prostitution.[19]

Perhaps, ironically, the early twentieth-century social hygienists who campaigned against VD were right to call it a "social disease"—but not in the way they thought. Indeed, this last bit of historical data, about the ways STIs have been linked with and even personified as "deviant" persons or groups, is particularly instructive for how we might read information about STIs with empirical justice and hermeneutic competency. STIs as we have framed and continue to frame them feed the worst features of our social structures and our social selves. As long as we treat them as afflictions of a vicious other, we allow STIs to feed our own vices of prejudice, domination, apathy, and greed.

In large part because of their long-standing association with otherness, STIs are also weapons of power-based oppression. Because of their direct connection to behaviors of which societies disapprove and would prefer not to discuss, STIs often serve as an excuse for moral and material neglect—a sort of world kin of cosmic justice whereby those who misbehave are appropriately stricken, obviating any cause to engage with them or attend to their needs. STIs also act as a metric by which to define out-groups as other, a means to justify ill-treatment of underclasses. Sometimes they are the means of ill-treatment itself, as was the case with the Tuskegee syphilis study. Other times, the out-group is itself pathologized. Poor people, women, and racial and sexual minorities are mapped onto pathogens: syphilis has the body of a beautiful woman, as in many World War II–era propaganda posters; AIDS is the "gay disease."

Discourses of sexual otherness, as well as a lack of frank and accurate public discourse about sex, sexuality, and sexual health, also stymie the successful management of STIs. The consistent portrayal of STIs as the fruits of immoral or antisocial sexual behavior, combined with the view that sex is a fundamentally private matter, means that openly discussing the ubiquity of sex and its attendant risks has not been considered appropriate for polite conversation or thorough public discussion. This is particularly true for adolescents—a group for whom solid education and preventive care is especially important.[20] It is also true even between sexual partners, since "the kind of communication that is necessary to explore a partner's sexual history, establish STD risk status, and plan for protection against STDs is made difficult by the taboos that surround sex and sexuality."[21] Such taboos also affect health care providers. Rates of STI screening in primary care settings are far below where they ought to be, a fact that can be at least partly attributed to providers' lack of comfort asking about their patients' sex lives—or, conversely, patients' discomfort with discussing their sex lives with their providers, especially if they worry that the details of their sex lives will cause providers to stigmatize them.[22] Furthermore, at least until quite recently, medical training has offered relatively little about sexuality, since it "continues to reflect the predominant opinion of society that sexual health issues are private issues."[23]

Pushing back against this lack of discourse is important, because any risk-management strategies are only as effective as the correctness and consistency of their implementation. Teaching interventions, like mechanical and biomedical ones, also depends on this correctness and consistency. A program that is effective in a study will do little good if it is not actually implemented and funded. Public health approaches that recognize the multifactorial nature of STI risk, the reasons people may avoid preventive measures or treatment, and the reasons people engage in relatively higher-risk activities (multiple partners, serial monogamy, casual sex, and so on) can help lower transmission rates, especially if they focus on making services more easily available to the people who need them most.

Thus, any adequate moral account of STIs must, minimally, meet two criteria. First, it must facilitate open conversations about sexuality, sexual risks, and STI status. In practical terms, this means normalizing regular testing, disclosure of STI status, and use of appropriate preventive measures. Second, it must understand that disparities in social stigma and in access to and quality of care are also fundamentally moral issues.

In what follows, I outline a model for thinking about the ethics of STIs that meets these criteria. In this chapter, I argue that the mishnaic treatment of ritual impurity offers a promising model for thinking about STIs. The Mishnah, as I demonstrate below, treats ritual impurity as a form of social contagion—an undesirable but unavoidable and manageable consequence of desirable forms of social interaction. Understanding STIs in similar terms, I argue, will do a great deal to reduce stigma and shame and to help us manage STI risk in an effective and humane manner. I discuss the phenomenon of ritual impurity as it appears in the Mishnah, using the Zavim tractate as a case study through which to focus on the aspects of ritual impurity most applicable to STI management. Ultimately, I argue, the rabbis of the Mishnah not only offer us a model for thinking about the ethics of sex and public health; they also offer us a way to think more broadly about the ethics of risk. Crip theory, as I argued in chapter 2, shows us that acknowledging, managing, and honestly living with risk is crip and queer. Mishnaic purity discourse shows us a system by which such practice is also deeply virtuous.

Leaky Lessons: What We Can Learn from Mishnah Zavim

If the dominant social frameworks through which we currently approach STI transmission are unhelpful at best and actively harmful at worst, what other frameworks are available? One promising framework, I argue, lies in the ways tannaitic texts explore questions of ritual impurity, which, for the rabbis of the Mishnah, functions as a form of contagion that is an undesirable but ultimately inevitable consequence of social intercourse, which, in turn, is desirable in its own right in spite of its risks. Impurity in the Mishnah is a morally significant category but not in the ways we might expect. It was, as Mira Balberg argues, a constant in the daily lives of those who inhabit the rabbinic world. This constant presence of impurity conditioned how one understood the nature of the body and the effect of bodily encounters upon daily life in terms of this ever-present possibility of transmission. Individuals and communities must mitigate impurity in ways that are attentive to its characteristics. Furthermore, within the class of ritual impurity, there exist numerous types and degrees of impurity, each of which has different consequences and different mitigation protocols. And the Mishnah neither trivializes the consequences of transmitting impurity, nor does it treat impurity as something that is alien or shameworthy. The moral implications of ritual impurity do not lie in the simple matter of being or not being impure; rather, they lie in the way persons discipline themselves so that they may best mitigate the consequences of being social actors in a world where impurity is an inevitable consequence of social interaction. And the moral models we can derive from this account of ritual impurity are far better frameworks for an ethics of sexual health than Western history on the matter has largely offered thus far.

Here, I examine selected texts from Mishnah Zavim, which deals with irregular genital discharges, or zivah, as type cases. Zavim displays several key traits that offer especially useful models for thinking through contemporary matters of sexual health. Three of these traits concern the character of ritual impurity itself. First, in Zavim, as with other comparable texts, ritual impurity is ubiquitous and ultimately unavoidable. This is a critical corrective to regnant depictions of STIs as diseases of the other, for the Mishnah gives us a picture of socially transmitted contagion as everyone's risk and everyone's concern. Second, Zavim, again like other comparable texts, differentiates between multiple categories and subcategories of impurity, each requiring its own procedures of diagnosis and treatment. Here, too, it offers a critical corrective to regnant accounts of STIs as monolithic, such that one is either infected or "clean" and in which one particularly frightening infection stands in for all possible STIs (think, for example, of how "VD" nearly always meant "syphilis" for much of the twentieth century). Third, Zavim distinguishes between what I call the *absolute virulence* and *absolute severity* and the *contextual virulence* and *contextual severity* of different types of impurity, understanding that while one type of impurity might affect more overall ritual functions and have more overall routes of transmission than others, it does not always follow that it is the greatest concern in any given circumstance. This account offers a framework for understanding similar distinctions within STI epidemiology: while one STI may be more absolutely virulent than others, it does not follow that it is the greatest public health concern in all contexts.

Zavim's next key trait deals with the ways those who inhabit an impurity-laden world interact with one another. Zavim's world is one in which intimate human interaction is inevitable, one of social beings who touch each other in multiple ways. It assumes that people will have regular physical interactions with each other: engaging in household or workplace tasks that cause them to touch, shift, or lean on one another, touching or moving shared items that others will also touch or move, and simply sharing physical space in proximity. While all these interactions involve rabbinically recognized routes of impurity transmission, such interactions are nevertheless inevitable and even desirable. This is a deeply important corrective to a regnant sexual ethic that dichotomizes "safe" and "risky" sex and claims that any sex that seems to risk STI transmission is not worth the risks of doing. But Zavim reminds us that almost all social intimacy carries some risk and models a way of valuing that intimacy while explicitly acknowledging its potential to do harm.

Finally, Zavim, like nearly all classical rabbinic texts, treats its subject matter in exhaustive and explicit detail. For the purposes of sexual ethics, however, it is particularly important that the subject matter that Zavim and other purity texts treat in this exhaustive detail concerns socially transmitted contagion. STIs have historically been treated and often continue to be treated euphemistically, through a thick miasma of shame, stigma, and embarrassment. But rabbinic discourse about ritual impurity models a way of talking about social contagion that can clear this miasma through its sheer barrage of detail and, even more importantly, through its willingness to treat that very detail as a subject that is at once worthy of serious thought and yet is so mundane and so unremarkable as to be all in a day's discussion.

All together, these key traits explicitly encourage an ethic of self-awareness cultivated through practices of regular self-examination, something that is characteristic of mishnaic impurity discourse more generally and that has clear implications for STI management. Virtuous rabbinic agents build their daily routines around practices of examination meant to foster self-control and self-awareness. Rabbinic subjects must then interpret the results of these examinations, usually with either direct or indirect expert aid, to determine whether it is likely they have contracted some form of impurity that requires mitigation.[24] This sort of self-examination is considered virtuous for everyone, not just those who engage in some sort of high-impurity-risk behavior.[25] Self-inventory is not a behavioral sin tax levied against those who are socially or occupationally lax; it is a mental and behavioral ideal to be striven for. In fact, the ubiquitous character of impurity and the subsequent practical need for regular self-examination are, as Balberg argues, best understood as an opportunity to cultivate self-examination and self-awareness as components of a virtuous character in their own right.[26] In other words, that a particular kind of contagion is practically unavoidable for all social actors means that the management strategies necessitated by that contagion also teach us how to be better social actors more generally.

The worth of the Mishnah's emphasis on socially embedded self-awareness and regular self-examination should become readily apparent when we consider the fact that a significant contributor to STI transmission is simple ignorance of one's STI status.[27] Perversely, a potential partner who discloses a known and well-managed infection may appear to present a greater risk than a potential partner who assumes or claims to be infection-free but has no concrete information to back up that assertion.[28] Stigma helps perpetuate ignorance, which then, in a vicious cycle, further perpetuates stigma; the less we know, the more we fill that vacuum with the narratives of STIs as diseases of the other that we are already used to.

That must change. We should encourage knowing more, something that cannot happen if we dread to discover that we might have an STI because we know so little about them and think of them as marks of social shame and moral disgrace. The Mishnah's emphasis on socially embedded self-knowledge and self-examination offers an alternative vision. The specific traits of Zavim's treatment of impurity—the ubiquity of impurity, the importance of a fine-grained differential diagnosis among many subtypes of impurity, the distinction among contextual and absolute virulence and severity, the recognition of the many types of transmission-risking intimate social interactions that a person might experience on a given day, and the overarching practice of talking about contagion in exhaustive detail—provide the beginnings of a blueprint for achieving that vision.

Ubiquity

When we live in a world in which we are constantly, materially interacting with other embodied actors, contagion of one kind or another among those actors is ultimately inevitable. To treat contagion as something only experienced by morally suspect others is to fundamentally misunderstand the ways we exist in physical and social space.

The Mishnah, however, not only recognizes this ubiquity but predicates its entire understanding of ritual impurity upon it. Tannaitic literature follows the Pentateuch in recognizing two broad categories of impurity, ritual and moral, and it bases its categories and sources of impurity on those enumerated there.[29] In both the Pentateuch and in the tannaitic literature, ritual impurity is largely unavoidable, temporary, and communicable and not to be confused with moral defilement. But while in the Bible contracting ritual impurity is a discrete event, in rabbinic literature impurity resides in diffuse and often imperceptible webs of transmission.[30] Someone who enters one of these webs may not realize that they have done so until well after the fact, if at all. Thus, the rabbinic world is one in which impurity is ubiquitous, to the point where even zivah, a form of impurity that by definition results from an *abnormal* penile discharge, is treated as though it were matter-of-fact and commonplace.

Rabbinic discourse thus presumes that the transmission of impurity is what could be called a "known unknown." One may not know whether, at any given time, they have contracted a given impurity, but they must always assume the possibility of such contraction in any given encounter. Practically speaking, this means that one must assume that possibility most of the time, because the rabbinic world is also one that is populated by social beings who interact with each other and touch each other in a variety of ways. Even as the rabbis extend the biblical mechanisms of transmission to include indirect physical contact, they also assume that the average person will regularly act in ways that open them up to these expanded mechanisms of transmissions. Intimate human interaction, for the rabbis, necessarily places one within multiple webs of impurity, but it is also simply inevitable. And this inevitability offers an important corrective to regnant views of STIs as singular events that denote moral failings. For if contagion is a constant presence—even if most STIs are not, unlike ritual impurity, precisely default—then shaming and shunning those who contract it becomes far more difficult.

To better understand the inevitability of ritual impurity, consider some of the situations described in Zavim 3:2:

> If [a zav and a pure person] were closing or opening a door [together], [they are both impure.] But the Sages say: only if this one closed it, and the other one opened it.
>
> If one brought the other up from a pit, Rabbi Yehudah said: [they are both impure] only when the one who is pure lifts out the one who is impure.
>
> If they were knotting ropes together, the Sages say: [they are both impure] only if one pulled his way and the other pulled his own way.
>
> If they were weaving [together], whether they were standing or sitting, or if they were grinding grain together, Rabbi Shimon declares the one who is pure to be fully pure, unless they were grinding with a hand-held millstone.
>
> If they were unloading a donkey, or loading it, when the load is heavy the pure one is impure, but when the load is light, he remains pure.
>
> But in all such cases they are pure enough for the members of the congregation, and impure for the purposes of eating terumah.

This passage lists several examples of physical interactions through which it is possible to transmit zivah. The passage thus takes for granted two things: first, that it is very easy to enter a zivah-transmission web and, second, that people will regularly engage in activities that bring them into this web. In the examples described here, the inevitability of physical interaction that might transmit zivah is underscored by the mundane character of each situation. Any of these interactions could quite plausibly occur during the course of a normal day in a preindustrial society. Furthermore, five of the six examples—one person lifting another out of a pit, knotting ropes together, weaving together, grinding grain together, or loading or unloading a pack animal—could easily be a regular part of day-to-day subsistence work. Thus, not only the normal course of social relations more broadly but also the normal course of economic relations dictate that these interactions are bound to occur and to occur regularly.

The enumeration of the common, quotidian, subsistence-related actions through which anyone can enter a zivah-transmission web have clear import for thinking about STIs, which have usually been diseases of "them," the other. To the extent communities have considered STIs to be of concern it has been couched in terms of their being a threat originating from "them." Along those lines, while STIs might be considered the "default" status for "them," they were a terrifying deviation from the norm for "us." Among "us," the contraction of an STI would be a shameful, singular event, a personal and social crisis resulting from engaging in unspeakable, antisocial forms of interaction.

In the Mishnah, however, impurity is ubiquitous. Not only is it not the stigmatized domain of the other; it is something that the rabbis—the social and ritual elite and the assumed "we" of the text's narrative voice—assume to be true of themselves. Impurity isn't just not something that happens to the "wrong" sort; it's something that the most learned, most righteous figures within the textual world are constantly navigating.[31] As a result, the Mishnah "presents [impurity] as the daily and ongoing concern of *everyone* [within the Jewish community], even of persons who are not currently impure or known to have had contact with a source of impurity."[32] And, in the passage from Zavim I treat here, the actions through which one risks contracting zivah are not clandestine misdeeds but rather mundane, subsistence activities that everyone not only can do but must do. All this reduces the extent to which it is possible to shame someone for having contracted impurity—after all, one cannot render a person alien for something that is recognized to be everyone's problem and everyone's concern.

That impurity is default, then, means that it cannot be an occasion for panic. Nor can it, in and of itself, be an occasion for shunning or disdain. While lax or inappropriate engagement with the default reality of impurity can be and is occasion for disdain, as is the case with the amei ha'arets ("people of the land"), nonrabbinic Jews who are castigated for their assumed carelessness regarding impurity, the risk of contracting impurity or the fact of having contracted impurity itself is so accepted and commonplace as to be nearly unremarkable.[33] As I discuss further below, this characteristic therefore makes the strategies for managing impurity similarly unremarkable. Impurity is an unavoidable consequence of certain types of social intercourse. It requires awareness and management, but it is no cause for alarm.

The parallels here are not perfect. Generally speaking, STIs are not default or unavoidable in the same ways that ritual impurity was default for the rabbis of the Mishnah, although herpes simplex virus (HSV), whose combined global prevalence between HSV-1 (primarily oral) and HSV-2 (primarily genital, though either virus can infect either area) is estimated at 78 percent—likely higher, since many people with herpes do not know that they are infected—is an exception.[34] But, while STI rates can and should be drastically reduced, there is no way to engage in partnered sex that completely eliminates any risk of STIs—a reality acknowledged by the recent shift in emphasis from a language of "safe sex" to that of "safer sex."[35] The range of different types of infection, some of which are transmitted through fluids and others of which are easily transmitted through skin-to-skin contact; the rapidly evolving character of bacteria and viruses; the variability of human cultural norms, values, and sexual preferences; and the simple fact that humans are error-prone beings mean that STIs will always be a moving target. So while STIs are not default like ritual impurity, they are like ritual impurity in that they cannot, at a collective level, be completely avoided, only managed. And it is by attending to and internalizing STIs' collective ubiquity that we can make the first step toward making them discussable without shame. Recognizing this is not to encourage fatalism—it is not inevitable that any given person will contract one or more STIs, and it is important that individuals and communities take reasonable steps toward prevention. Yet ironically, these reasonable steps will remain inaccessible to many if we continue to treat STIs as a problem only affecting a blighted few.

Differential Diagnoses

Social contagion is ubiquitous, but it is not monolithic, even if we are tempted to treat it as such. Rather, there are many kinds and degrees of social contagion that may pose greater or lesser risks depending on context. Regnant STI discourse has generally failed to account for this, treating a variety of STIs as a single crisis, but it is something the Mishnah explicitly recognizes. Integral to the system of management we find in Mishnah Zavim are complex processes of diagnosis of impurity and various programs of response whose particulars depend on the particulars of a given diagnosis. A proper differential diagnosis requires one to determine *impurity status* (whether someone is impure), *type of impurity* (to which biblical source one's impurity can be traced), and *degree of impurity* (how severe one's impurity is and thus whether one must perform the full biblical purification ritual or an abbreviated and less onerous one). These determinations, as we shall see, affect not only how one must treat one's case of impurity but how virulent that case is. Impurity, in short, is not monolithic. Not all impurities are alike, and not all impurities, even within a given type of impurity, are to be treated the same way. This stands, as we shall see, in sharp contrast to prevailing attitudes about STIs, according to which one is either "clean" or not and in which the most notorious STI within one's particular social context comes to stand for all STIs. The Mishnah's process of differential diagnosis reminds us that social contagion is not so easily reducible.

This complex, multifactorial process of differential diagnosis is a mishnaic innovation. Biblical zivah, as described in Leviticus 15:2–15, occurs when anyone has a nonseminal discharge that either oozes from or blocks his penis. (A seminal discharge causes ḳeri, a different, less severe type of impurity.) This person is impure, transmits impurity by directly touching, lying on, sitting on, leaning on, spitting on, carrying, or being carried upon various persons or objects, and is liable for a purification ritual in which he waits seven days, purifies himself by washing his clothes and body in "living" or flowing water, and makes an offering to a priest. There, one is either a zav or one is not. Zavim 1:1, by contrast, adds qualifications of volume, repetition, and timing to determine whether someone with a genital discharge is a *zav gamur*, or a "true zav"—that is, one who conveys impurity in all the ways described in Leviticus 15:2–15 and is thus liable for the full purification ritual:

> If a man sees a single discharge of zivah: Bet Shammai say, he is like a woman who watches day against day; but Bet Hillel say, he is like one who has had a seminal emission.
>
> If he saw one [emission of discharge], and it ceased on the second day, and on the third day he sees two [emissions of discharge], or one issue with the volume of two:
>
> Bet Shammai say, he is a true zav. But Bet Hillel says, he renders impure what he lies or sits upon, and he must immerse in the mikveh, but he is exempt from an offering.

Rabbi Eliezer ben Yehudah said: Bet Shammai agree that in that case, he is
not a true zav, but they differ regarding the one who sees two emissions, or
one emission with the volume of two, whose emissions ceased on the second
day and who saw a single emission on the third day:
Bet Shammai say, *this* one is a true zav. But Bet Hillel say, he renders
impure what he lies or sits upon, and he must immerse in the ritual bath, but
he is exempt from an offering.

This mishnah thus establishes several degrees of zivah, each requiring a different degree of remedy. Further, by comparing a minimal quantity of zivah
discharge to a normal seminal emission, this mishnah reiterates the biblical
distinction between zivah impurity and ḳeri (seminal) impurity. ḳeri is also
an impurity-causing genital emission, but it is a different type of impurity
than is zivah, although it may be used as a point of comparison with certain
degrees of zivah. While any discharge from the penis causes some impurity,
the discharge must be of a particular type (abnormal and oozing or forming
a blockage), add up to a certain volume, and repeat within a certain amount
of time to qualify as the true zivah, conveying impurity in the manner described and requiring the full ablutions and ritual offering stipulated in the
passage from Leviticus. Thus, impurity status (whether a person has contracted ritual impurity of any kind) is distinguished from type of impurity
(which biblical source caused the impurity) and degree of impurity (which
deals with differences between particular impurities' severities, virulences,
and prescribed remedies).

This stands in stark contrast to the way we have tended to treat STIs as
a singular entity, effectively reducing diagnosis to impurity status: one is
either "clean" or "infected," and we make little or no distinction among different pathogens, infections, or syndromes. Indeed, one STI may become
metonymic for STIs in general: early and mid-twentieth-century campaigns
against "venereal disease," for example, were in fact overwhelmingly campaigns against syphilis, even though gonorrhea was much more prevalent.
Such a monolithic view of STIs, however, is both medically and socially in-
accurate, as there are many different infections, some viral, some bacterial,
and some fungal, which occur at different rates in different social contexts,
paralleling the Mishnah's category of type of impurity. Furthermore, different stages of a given infection may pose different risks of transmission
and have different symptoms or lack thereof—something I discuss in more

detail below—and require different protocols for treatment, testing, and social conduct, paralleling the category of degree of impurity. For example, when herpes is not causing an outbreak, it is nearly impossible to determine whether one is infected, and one's risk of transmitting it to a partner is reduced. If one knows one has herpes, one might take suppressive medication to reduce the risk of an outbreak and to reduce one's risk of transmitting it. When one has an outbreak, however, one must treat the sore and refrain from bringing it into contact with partners.

In addition to attending to the physical and temporal details of the discharge itself, a proper diagnostic process must attend to the circumstances of exchange with the physical and social environment at the time of the precipitating event. Zavim 2:2 demonstrates this attention as it addresses the process of examination for a suspected zav:

> There are seven lines along which a zav, the nature of whose discharge is yet undetermined, is examined: concerning food, drink, what he has carried, whether he has jumped, whether he has been sick, what he has seen, and what he has thought about: did he have sexual thoughts before he saw [an arousing sight], or did he see [the arousing sight] before he had sexual thoughts?
>
> Rabbi Yehudah said: even if he saw beasts, wild animals, or birds going at each other, even if he saw the dyed garments of a woman.
>
> Rabbi Akiva said: even if he ate all he could eat, whether bad or pleasing, or drank any drink.
>
> They said to him: according to your logic, there would never be any zavim!
>
> He said to them: the future existence of zavim is not your problem!

This mishnah establishes that attentiveness to the circumstances of exchange are critical for establishing not just degree of impurity but even for establishing the more basic category of type of impurity. The processes of examination for a suspected zav described here are meant to rule out other potential causes of discharge, since otherwise it would be conceivable that the emission was something other than zivah. If, for example, it is possible that the suspected zav experienced some kind of stimulus that might have triggered a spontaneous ejaculation of semen, that may be enough to cast his status as a zav into doubt. Similarly, discharge could be explained as an incidental consequence of eating a certain food or taking a certain action—in any of these cases, the discharge "will be dismissed as incidental and not as an indication of a pathological condition."[36] Thus, the physical and temporal qualities of the discharge itself are not the only categories that are determinative of its ultimate character and consequence. The circumstances of the subject's exchange with their environment at the time of the precipitating event—where they were, what they perceived, what they thought about, with whom they interacted—all of these are also crucial data points for the diagnostician. STIs, too—the risks of contracting and transmitting them, as well as the risks of morbidity and mortality from them—are mediated both by people's circumstances of exchange or contraction and by their ongoing experiences after the initial exchange. Simply put, environment matters for social contagions, ritual impurity and STIs alike.

Contextual and Absolute Virulence and Severity

Accepting the variability of social contagion, and the fact that this variability is mediated by the circumstances under which contagion is transmitted, also means recognizing the fact that different contagions will have different levels of severity and different levels of virulence in different circumstances. This is certainly true of STIs. Different infections have different levels of virulence (the likelihood of spread and infection) and different levels of severity (how sick an infection makes one), but this is a point often underappreciated, even where the existence of diverse varieties of STI is recognized. Take, for example, the stigma surrounding herpes. There are two major strains of herpes simplex virus; HSV-1 is primarily oral and HSV-2 primarily genital, although either virus can colonize either area; both are transmitted through direct contact with the affected area or effluvia from an outbreak. Current estimates place HSV-1 prevalence in the United States at around 65 percent and HSV-2 prevalence in the US in individuals between the ages of fourteen and forty-nine at 15.5 percent.[37] Worldwide combined HSV-1 and HSV-2 prevalence is around 90 percent. This means that more people have herpes than do not.[38] And, outside of specific situations, such as when someone who is in labor has an outbreak and thereby risks transmitting the herpes infection to the infant, herpes is more of a nuisance than a genuine medical danger. Yet the stigma of herpes is incongruent with both its actual dangers (relatively small) and its prevalence (relatively large).

Accurate assessment of the implications of a given contagion therefore requires attending not only to the source's absolute virulence but also to the circumstances that affect its contextual virulence and to varying levels of severity. And here, once again, the Mishnah is instructive, for it extensively discusses exactly that, recognizing that different sources of impurity have varying levels of virulence and, to a much lesser extent, severity that are contextually mediated. In this context, severity indicates how intensive a purification ritual is required, while virulence refers to how transmissible the impurity is. Absolute virulence means the cumulative power of transmission of a given impurity outside of any particular case of transmission. It is determined by such factors as the total number of routes of transmission, the degree of secondary impurity communicated by contact with the source, and the directness of contact with the source required for transmission. Contextual virulence, by contrast, refers to a given impurity's power of transmission in a particular case.

Mishnaic purity discourse is quite careful to recognize multiple forms of impurity that have multiple levels of virulence and severity. As noted above, even within the relatively narrow realm of "impurities related to male genital discharge," the Mishnah recognizes two types of impurity and multiple degrees of impurity within those types, not all of which are of equal virulence and severity. The first chapter of Zavim is almost entirely devoted to distinguishing between a true zav, who is liable for the full purification ritual detailed in Leviticus 15 and who transmits impurity in all the ways described there, and someone who has a lesser degree of zivah impurity, is less contagious, and requires a less intensive purification ritual. It is, in other words, concerned with which types and degrees of male genital discharge impurities are more and less absolutely severe and absolutely virulent than others.

Outside of zivah-type impurities, the variety is even greater, and the question of varying levels of virulence is explicitly discussed in multiple places. The first chapter of Mishnah Kelim ranks sources according to their routes of contagion—the more routes of transmission, the more virulent the source. A *metsora* (someone with an impure skin condition) is a strong vector of impurity, while someone who has sex with a nidah (a menstruating woman) is a weaker vector.[39] People and objects can both be sources of impurity, and whether the initial source is a person or an object also affects its virulence: zivah discharge, and disembodied fluids from a zav have fewer possible routes of transmitting impurity than does a zav himself.[40] Further, there are intermediate levels of impurity and virulence at different stages in the purification

process (often a multiday affair): someone who has immersed to begin purification during the day but who will not be fully pure until nightfall may participate in some rituals afforded to the pure (eating tithes) but not in others
(eating foods that carry a higher level of consecration).[41] A metsora is one of
the strongest vectors of impurity, ranking behind only a corpse and a bone
fragment, but a metsora who has recovered and is waiting out their days of
purification is one of the weakest vectors.[42]

One significant factor in the contextual virulence of a given impurity is the
set of routes by which that impurity can be communicated. In the Mishnah,
each source of impurity has its own set of standardized routes; while there
is overlap among sources, a given source will be at least somewhat different
from others in terms of the set of routes by which it may transmit. Further,
the possible routes may vary depending on what the impurity is being transmitted to. Zivah, Zavim 2:4 tells us, has five possible routes of transmission:

> The zav conveys impurity in five ways, so that a person and their clothing are
> impure: to what he stands on, what he sits on, what he lies on, what he hangs
> on, and what he leans on.
>
>   And what he lies on conveys impurity to a person so that they in turn
> convey impurity to garments by standing, sitting, hanging, leaning, touching,
> or carrying.

The Mishnah goes on to specify zivah's routes of secondary transmission:
in addition to direct contact with a zav, a lesser degree of zivah impurity can
be spread by contact with something a zav lay upon, and that person in turn
communicates impurity (although a lesser degree of it) through one more
route than does the zav himself.[43]

Some sources have more absolute power to communicate impurity—that
is to say, they are more virulent—than others. M. Kelim 1:3–4 addresses the
zav's place in this hierarchy, ranking the zav as a more virulent source than a
number of others, even more than his own bodily fluids, but it ranks a zavah
(a woman with abnormal genital discharge), a metsora (someone with an
impure skin condition), a small bone fragment, and a corpse as more virulent
than a zav. This, combined with what we learn from Zavim 2:4 about the zav's
five modes of transmission and the graded impurity of those persons and objects to which zivah impurity is communicated, seems to tell us conclusively
that the zav is moderately contagious among other sources of impurity.

Zavim 4:6, however, complicates this ranking of virulence. It describes a hypothetical case in which a zav and pure food or drink are sitting in the pans of a balance scale. If the zav's weight causes the food to move, the food is thereby rendered impure:[44]

> If a zav were in one pan of a set of scales, and food or drink were in the second pan, they are impure; but if a corpse [were in the first pan], anything [in the second pan], save a person, remains pure.
>
> This is a case where greater stringency applies to a zav than to a corpse. But greater stringency is also applied to a corpse than to a zav. For a zav renders impure anything under him that is fit for lying or sitting on, such that it in turn renders persons and garments impure; he also conveys *madaf*-impurity [another term for indirect contact impurity] to whatever lies above him, such that it in turn conveys impurity to food and drink—impurity which a corpse does not covey.
>
> But greater stringency applies to a corpse, because a corpse conveys impurity by overhang, and it conveys seven days' worth of impurity—impurity which a zav does not convey.

This direct comparison to corpse impurity complicates a straightforward ranking of impurity sources in terms of their virulence. M. Kelim 1:4 ranks a corpse as the most absolutely virulent type of impurity because it can transmit impurity through "overhang" and makes anyone who touches it impure for seven days, which no other source can do. In other words, it is capable of transmitting a higher degree of impurity (seven-day) through a more indirect route of transmission than any other source. M. Zavim 4:6, however, points out that a zav can, depending on the circumstance, have greater contextual virulence than can a corpse. Even though a corpse can communicate impurity through more routes than can a zav, a zav can communicate impurity in a way a corpse cannot, by indirect contact to items that lie above him such that they can then contaminate food and drink. The general rule may be that the corpse is a more absolutely virulent type of impurity than the zav, but there are circumstances in which the zav has greater contextual virulence than the corpse. Different impurities, in short, have different traits, and those particular traits may be more helpful in understanding which source is a greater concern in a given situation than is an abstract ranking of virulence.

This variability—the fact that there can be no one "strongest" paradigm impurity—has important corrective implications for a culture that has historically subsumed all STIs into "the worst" one and then focused on that to the exclusion of others, for context also matters when analyzing the risks different STIs pose. While the Mishnah focuses largely on contextual versus absolute virulence, its logic can be extended to both virulence and severity in the case of STIs. Above, I discussed herpes, whose reputation is all out of proportion to its absolute severity. However, in a case where a person in labor has an outbreak and risks transmitting the infection to the newborn—a situation that can have very serious consequences for the baby—herpes takes on much higher contextual severity. Or take the case of HIV, which is among the most absolutely severe STIs known and also has fairly high absolute virulence. Untreated, it is almost invariably fatal, and it is also easily transmissible through blood and semen. However, contemporary antiretroviral treatment not only turns HIV into a chronic, manageable condition but also significantly reduces its virulence. Someone who has been on antiretroviral drugs long enough to bring their viral loads down to undetectable levels is, for most practical intents and purposes, no longer contagious.[45] Responsible use of barrier methods and prophylactic drugs lower the risk of infection even further. Thus, even though HIV has very high absolute severity and fairly high absolute virulence, its contextual severity and contextual virulence may in many cases be much lower.

By contrast to HIV, gonorrhea does not have high absolute severity: while it can lead to significant complications if left untreated, it is unlikely to be fatal.[46] Because it is a bacterial STI, however, it is one of the commonplace conditions whose treatment is increasingly affected by the growing problem of antibiotic resistance.[47] Although most people manage to clear even drug-resistant gonorrhea on their own, reinfection is common. One of the easiest ways to spread drug-resistant gonorrhea is by way of fellatio, which, ironically enough, is reputed to be a safer sex practice through which one can reduce one's risk of contracting HIV. So, in certain contexts—communities where HIV rates are well under control and people have access to effective treatment—gonorrhea certainly has greater contextual virulence and may well have greater contextual severity and thus be a greater overall risk than HIV.

Closely attending to this complex variation makes it much harder to turn STIs into a monolith; it also complicates any knee-jerk fear of STIs as unmitigated disasters and of those who might have them as terrifying plague carriers. Dealing with STI risk, like many other social risks, means dealing with context-dependent variables. Different STIs are one set of factors that can change the specific variables one must deal with in any given circumstance. Thinking well about those variables forces one to be more closely attentive to context generally—an important skill for any social actor.

Regular Intimate Interaction

One especially pernicious feature of regnant STI discourse is how it figures STIs as a natural consequence of specific kinds of sexual interaction—usually, penetrative sexual acts between people who are not married to one another. This works both to stigmatize people who are assumed to have STIs and to participate in these acts, making testing, treatment, and social support less accessible to them, and to obscure equally viable routes of STI transmission that do not fall into this category, causing others to erroneously assume that they are not at risk.

The Mishnah, however, recognizes that people engage in many forms of physically and socially intimate interaction throughout the day and that the forms of contact that matter most for transmitting contagion are not necessarily the most direct or obvious ones. Nor are the sorts of intimate interactions that are inevitable throughout day-to-day social life always planned, desired, or cooperative, although they often are. Indeed, these forms of contact may be desired or even needed for reasons that have nothing to do with their potential to transmit impurity. Zavim 3:3, for example, mainly consists of a discussion of quotidian situations that are potential vectors for transmitting impurity by heseṭ, or shift:

> If a zav and one who is pure sat together in a large boat—
>   What is a large boat? Rabbi Yehudah says, any that cannot be destabilized by the weight of one person—
>   or if they sat on a plank, or a stool, or on a bed-frame, or on a beam, where these are secured; or if they were in a stable tree, or in a stable booth, or on a heavy ladder, or on an Egyptian ladder secured by a nail, or a gangway, or a rafter, or a door, where they have been plastered with clay, even if they only went up one end, the pure person and his garments remain pure.

Impurity is transmitted by way of heseṭ when a pure person and an impure person share some kind of platform, and the impure person indirectly causes the pure person to move. Thus, in all the cases discussed here, the shared platform is presumed to be stable enough that any normal movements made

by the zav will be insufficient to cause the pure person to move. This is as opposed to the situations described in Zavim 3:1—of which this discussion is a
continuation—all of which are identical save for the fact that the platforms
are unsecured or, in the case of the boat, small enough that one person's
movement will shift those with whom he shares it. Thus, perhaps counterin-
tuitively, the fact of shared space—even intimately, closely shared space—is
not the most salient factor in whether impurity is transmitted. Rather, it is
one specific sort of interaction among many—whether a shared platform
is unstable enough that the zav's movement translates to the pure person—
that determines whether impurity is communicated in these situations.

Thus far, all the interactions described in this mishnah are, like the cases
in 3:2 (treated in the discussion of the ubiquity of contagion, above), at least
neutral and often cooperative. The end of the Mishnah, however, seems to
abruptly shift focus to an adversarial interaction, asking what would occur if
a pure person and a zav were to engage in fisticuffs: "If a pure person strikes
an impure person, he remains pure. If an impure person strikes a pure person,
the pure person becomes impure, since if the pure person pulled back, the
impure person would then fall." Here, the Mishnah considers the outcome
of two possible permutations of a physical altercation between a pure person and a zav. If a pure person were to strike a zav, the pure person would
remain pure, despite the fact that to hit someone is necessarily to touch them.
If, on the other hand, the zav were to strike the pure person, the pure person would become impure. So, again, the most intuitively obvious mode of
interaction—in this case, the direct physical contact of hitting—is not the
mechanism of transmission. Rather, the rabbis assume that anyone who is
on the receiving end of a blow will automatically pull back from the force of
the blow for the sake of self-preservation. As a result, the zav causes the pure
person to shift his weight, thus communicating impurity by midras, that is,
by leaning on the pure person.

The inclusion of a bout of fisticuffs within a group of otherwise neutral
or even cooperative interactions demonstrates the Mishnah's expansive
understanding of the sorts of intimate interactions that are likely and even
inevitable within the course of day-to-day life. A person will be in physical
proximity to and engage in physical interactions of many kinds with many
different people, at least some of whom are likely to be in a state of impurity,
throughout the course of any given day. Not all those interactions may be

pleasant or desirable, and some may even be damaging, but all of them are part of the universe of social interaction and therefore bear consideration. Furthermore, even within a specific encounter, there are multiple subtypes of interaction that may occur, only some of which are salient to the question of whether impurity has been transmitted. The salient subtypes of interaction are not necessarily those that are most intuitively obvious—indeed, they are equally likely to be those types of interaction that one may not even consciously register as a form of interaction.

Once again, the Mishnah corrects regnant STI discourse by reminding us that everyone engages in behavior that is a potential transmission risk. This behavior may be desirable or necessary for reasons that are entirely orthogonal to that risk—like the physical, social, and emotional pleasures of sex, which are valuable in their own right, or the social and economic needs met through sex work—or it may be entirely unplanned and unintentional or even violent, as is, unfortunately, sexual assault. It also reminds us that the range of intimate interactions that pose transmission risks is far wider than we assume. Just because an infection is sexually transmissible, for example, does not mean that sexual acts are the only ways of transmitting it. I mentioned the near-universal prevalence of herpes above; part of the reason for this is that HSV-1—which, again, is primarily associated with oral herpes but which can also colonize the genitals—is transmissible not just by sex but by social pleasantries like a kiss on the cheek from a friend or relative. HIV, similarly, is transmissible by any route that involves the exchange of blood or breastmilk.

Even within the universe of sexual acts that risk STI transmission, some acts, like oral sex, are often treated as negligible STI risks. This is, in fact, true for some STIs but not all of them. The risks of HIV transmission from oral sex are small unless one or more of the participants has open cuts or sores in their mouth or on their genitals. But oral sex carries much more significant risks of transmitting HPV or gonorrhea than it does of HIV. In the case of the zav striking the pure person, the transmission comes not as a result of the interaction we'd intuitively expect—the contact of the strike itself—but from the less obvious fact of the zav causing the pure person to shift their weight. Similarly, in the two STI cases above, the greatest infection risk comes not from the acts we'd expect—penetrative sex (in which, furthermore, the transmission risk of those STIs whose primary vector is fluids is easily mitigated by using a condom)—but from the ones we're less likely to consider.

The case of the zav striking the pure person also demonstrates that contagion is one of many possible risks that we might encounter in our social lives and that it is perfectly reasonable to prioritize—consciously or not—other risks over and sometimes against those of contagion. The pure person contracts impurity by way of the impure person's leaning on them, something that happens because the pure person moves back to avoid the force of the zav's punch. That is to say, the pure person contracted zivah because they automatically and understandably prioritized avoiding the risk of getting hit over and against the risk—regardless of whether they knew their assailant was a zav—of contracting impurity.

We need to be able to understand, similarly, that STIs are some of many risks sexually active and potentially sexually active people encounter. It's true that there are some sexual practices that, all other things being equal, carry higher STI risks than others. But it doesn't follow that those who engage in those practices are not making conscious and careful choices about risk management. They may be carefully weighing priorities. Perhaps they acknowledge a heightened STI risk and, while taking appropriate steps to manage that where possible, have concluded that the risks of not engaging in those sexual practices—lack of sexual fulfillment, loss of valued community, loss of cultural expression, and so on—outweigh that heightened STI risk. These risks may not be as blatant as the risk of being struck by an assailant, but they can be equally damaging. Further, when someone who might appear to be taking serious sexual risks is part of a marginalized community, they may correctly recognize control of their sexual behavior as a potential mechanism of oppression. They may, in addition to wanting to avoid the pain of sexual restriction in and of itself, decide that the risk of sexual restriction as a political lever outweighs the risk of sexually transmitted infection. Or it may be that instead of being thoughtlessly risky, the actor is operating out of ignorance, because pursuing accurate information about sexual health and the resources to engage in safer sex practices opens one up to the danger of that same political control, as well as to the pain of shaming and condescension.

Exhaustive Detail: The Moral Power of Infodumping

It is precisely the ways in which control of sexuality and discourses of risk are wielded as tools of oppression that make the final feature of rabbinic impurity discourse so critical for interrupting it. While the features of Zavim's discussion of ritual impurity all provide important correctives to regnant treatments of STIs, perhaps the most important feature of Zavim, and of classical rabbinic discourse in general, is that it treats its subject matter in a levelheaded and intensely detailed way. Exhaustive—one might even say, ad nauseum—discussion of the finest details of a matter is characteristic of most classical rabbinic text; indeed, in colloquial English, to say a discussion is "Talmudic" is to say it is guilty of hairsplitting and hyperfocusing on the smallest and most incidental details.[48] But while the "Talmudic" epithet is often meant disparagingly, it is precisely this matter-of-fact and extensive hyperfocus on the details that constitutes a powerful moral technology for addressing matters like social contagion. For in doing so, it neutralizes the power of silence to perpetuate shame and stigma.

The fact that impurity takes multiple forms, each with its own routes of primary and secondary transmission, means that the encounter with impurity in the social world of the Mishnah is understood to be a constant. Thus, the Mishnah "presents [impurity] as the daily and ongoing concern of *everyone*, even of persons who are not currently impure or known to have had contact with a source of impurity."[49] As I have noted, this destigmatizes the contraction of impurity. Now I go one step further: the recognition of impurity's default status, and its resulting destigmatization, means that impurity is a thing about which it is possible to talk freely.

Open discussion of a matter is a critical step toward understanding it. Discussion allows the collection and comparison of relevant data and, consequently, the pooling of knowledge; it allows multiple minds to work on contextualizing and analyzing that data and multiple bearers of expertise to correct their own and each other's errors. Even beyond that, however, discussing something gives a name to it, makes it familiar, and tames it. Something unspeakable can be weaponized, and its victims made powerless to confront it directly. If, however, that thing can be discussed out in the open, there is a greater chance to defuse its impact. Those who need help managing that thing have the opportunity to stop hiding.

Making impurity normal and therefore discussable is the Mishnah's insight about how to *understand* and *conceptualize* social contagion; its emphasis on self-examination and self-awareness is its insight about how to *respond* to social contagion. Put another way, by making social contagion discussable, the Mishnah also makes it *actionable*. Having emphasized self-examination and self-awareness, the Mishnah goes on to offer a concrete prescription for the *sorts of action* it has now made possible. As mishnaic impurity discourse shows us, one way to manage something that is so widespread as to be unavoidable is to make it also unremarkable. To manage something, a community must be able to analyze it, discuss it, and understand that it is everyone's risk and everyone's concern. Rabbinic purity discourse thus models an account of STIs that takes them and their public health implications seriously without resorting to fearmongering or shaming. Impurity's constant presence in mishnaic discourse means that it is normalized but never allowed to fade from the collective consciousness. Along these lines, keeping discourse about sexual health status a constant presence in social interaction can normalize STI risk without trivializing it, in turn creating a communal climate that encourages subjects to cultivate the appropriate attention to their sexual health.

In short, the Mishnah reminds us that social contagion is complex. Dealing with it well requires us to reason about it, to talk about it, to make the discussion of its complexities as ubiquitous as the contagion itself. And by forcing us to think about the fine (and, yes, sometimes boring) details of social contagion, the Mishnah gives us a mode of reasoning about it that makes it much more difficult for us to default to shame, silence, and panic.

5. BDSM

Risk, Pleasure, and Polymorphous Community

IF STIS ARE ONE avenue through which all sexual actors encounter risks, sought after or not, the set of sexual practices encompassed by the labels BDSM and, more broadly, kink are an arena in which sexual actors deliberately seek out risk as an integral part of their practice.

As with STIs, BDSM represents a space in which the public, social, and communal dimensions of sexual interaction become apparent. In the case of STIs, this is because of their clear relationships to public health. In the case of BDSM, however, this is because a significant amount of BDSM activity occurs in public, communal spaces by design. Practitioners meet one another online as well as in "meatspace," and they gather at organized "play parties" usually overseen by a "dungeon monitor," meet-and-greet events called "munches" (during which no sex occurs), and skill-building classes and demonstrations to meet partners, enact "scenes," and develop technical skills and become more trustworthy and adept players, under communal auspices and oversight.

The term *BDSM* is an amalgamation of the initialisms for "bondage and discipline," "dominance and submission," and "sadism and masochism." It covers a wide variety of practices, interests, and communities; what these all share in common is that they involve thinking with, acting out, ritualizing, and eroticizing a range of power dynamics, physical sensations, and mental states that transgress accepted sociosexual norms in some way. Characteristic practices include but are not limited to bondage, spanking, flogging or caning, sensory deprivation, and dominant/submissive relationships that may be limited to a given enacted scene or may extend as far as 24/7 master/ slave relationships. More contested, riskier practices include such 24/7 "total power exchange," as well as blood play and asphyxiation. As I use it in this book, the term *kink* covers a similar range; however, it is less clearly or necessarily focused on painful sensations or power relationships. I also use *kinky* or *kinksters* to describe individuals or groups of individuals, whereas *BDSM* refers to a set of practices or a subculture or community that is organized around those practices. Thus, as I use the terms here, all BDSM practitioners are kinky, but not all kinksters necessarily practice BDSM.

Organized BDSM is a community in the sense I have described in chapter 2. It is founded on a central, identity-generating shared affinity; its signature shared activities discipline members toward further development of that identity, and it does this in a way that is based in and draws out moral responsibilities toward the group and its members. What is notable about this community is that its central affinity is an acknowledged risk activity. And in this, it is not unlike the classical rabbinic bet midrash as it is rendered within its own textual universe. The rabbinic canon, over and over again, demonstrates a clear awareness that the activity of scriptural interpretation—the activity on which a sage's identity is based and through which the sage disciplines his entire way of being to fit a sagely ideal—is always fraught with social, moral, physical, and metaphysical risk. The stakes of participating in the bet midrash are high indeed, but the rewards are great, as well, as is only befitting for an activity that is understood, in universe, as no less than playing with divine word.

If the BDSM dungeon, like the rabbinic bet midrash, is an example of what I shall call a *risk-conditioned community*, it offers us a moral corrective, one that is implicit in some ways in the bet midrash but that is here drawn out explicitly, for the critique of community I also raised in chapter 2—that it often, perhaps by definition, fails to accommodate and indeed can flatten, suppress, or banish difference, especially sexual difference on the grounds that it is disruptive or even contrary to the collective identity and welfare. The bet midrash contains some implicit counterpressure to this, for part of the risk at the center of its identity is pitched and even verbally violent disputation of matters of interpretation; without a structural accommodation and affirmation of some level of difference, such disputation could not occur. Organized BDSM, however, takes this further, for its central affinity, in addition to being based in risk, is also fundamentally based in difference and even deviance. Organized BDSM is by definition a community of sexual divergents, of people whose sexual identities, experiences, understandings, and desires diverge from a hegemonic norm. In this, its very existence suggests that community cannot only accommodate sexual difference and diversity but that it is possible even to found community upon this basis.

BDSM culture thus models ways in which cohesive communities can accommodate sexual difference. At the same time, it is also instructive because of the ways it can reflect and reproduce pernicious social hierarchies. And here, too, it resembles aspects of rabbinic culture in uncanny ways. The rabbis (and, again, I am referring to the rabbis as they refer to themselves inside the text rather than to the historical rabbis) shared with today's organized kinksters a similarly liminal position in a complex hierarchy of power. The rabbis were members of a religious and ethnic minority living under imperial rule; at the same time, they figured themselves as elites and authorities among that minority. They both wielded power and suffered others wielding it over them. Kinksters, similarly, are sexual minorities whose practices are subject to a range of social and sometimes legal opprobrium. Yet the organized kink communities studied by the ethnographers Staci Newmahr and Margot Weiss, on whose accounts I rely heavily in this chapter, tended to be overwhelmingly white, middle- to upper-middle-class, heterosexually identified, and cisgender.

In various execution rituals, the rabbis appropriate the mechanics and the optics of Roman power, "adapt[ing] the form of Roman execution [in] an effort to adapt the language of power and, in doing so, to challenge it."[1] But in doing so, they also risk reproducing and eventually resembling their Roman oppressors. Likewise, BDSM's dynamics can militate simultaneously toward liberation and toward neoliberal capitalist reentrenchment. Even any one given scene can hold this simultaneous potential: as Weiss notes, "Particular SM scenes might, by making sex public, disrupt understandings of sex as private, of desire as asocial, offering practitioners and analysts a new vantage point on the contradictions of current social relations." But the very same scenes can also risk obscuring or destroying that very potential: "They might also, by reprivatizing sex, create possibilities for a reentrenchment of subjects within such power structures, especially those that bolster the class, race, and gender inequality that is justified through neoliberal rationalities."[2]

Both the rabbinic practices and organized BDSM scenes thus resist any kind of unidirectional reading of their politics or their ethic. Indeed, the most interesting features of BDSM communities and practices may lie not in the individual acts performed so much as they may lie in *how* the acts are performed and interpreted. In this way, BDSM culture bears yet another similarity to rabbinic culture: just as the most interesting and contemporarily fruitful moral insights of rabbinic texts are to be gleaned not from their simple subject matter but rather from the functions of that subject matter within the rabbinic world or from the formal features of the ways in which the subject matter is discussed, so too are the most fruitful moral insights about "alternative" sexual practices found not in the "subject matter" of the practices themselves but rather in the social work those practices do in context and in the ways in which those practices are organized and interpreted.[3]

In what follows, I explore the parallels between rabbinic textual play and BDSM sexual play in what we might think of as a two-act drama. In the first act, using readings of the classic Talmudic passage known as the *tanur shel akhnai* (Oven of Akhnai) and of Staci Newmahr's and Margot Weiss's pivotal anthropologies of organized BDSM communities, I establish the rabbinic bet midrash (as portrayed within its own textual world) and the BDSM dungeon as parallel risk-conditioned communities, each of whose identity-generating affinity is a commitment to a set of activities that are acknowledged as both life-giving and as deeply and unavoidably risky. As a consequence of this centrality of risk, these communities socially, technically, and morally discipline members in ways that cultivate the skills necessary to manage that risk competently, wisely, and ethically. I then argue that because the BDSM dungeon is a habitus-building community whose existence is premised on sexual difference and diversity, it can help provide a model of a polymorphous, diverse community, one in which shared communal goals, disciplines, and interests do not quash or flatten but instead foster the flourishing of the sort of sexual and social diversity for whose moral value I argued in chapter 2.

In the second act, drawing strongly on Weiss's account, I trouble the picture I drew above by examining the ways in which organized BDSM fails to live up to its queerly diverse and communal ideal by reproducing many of the same hegemonies it seeks to resist or avoid. I make an analogy between these dynamics and the similarly troubled relationship with Roman techniques of execution the tannaitic rabbis evince in their own "execution play" in Mishnah Sanhedrin and the Mekhilta D'Rabbi Ishmael, drawing on Beth Berkowitz's reading of these texts. I then argue that the rabbis, along with marginalized BDSM players, especially Black women and disabled players, offer at least a partial corrective to some of these discontents. For while many of Weiss's subjects attempt to avoid the problematics of their practice by drawing a hard line between play and "real life," between semiprivate and fully public, the rabbis, like today's marginalized players, are keenly aware of the complex and fraught relationships between their practice and dominant power structures in which they are enmeshed. They understand all too well that text is not merely text, that play is not merely play, and that ritual can never be disentangled from the "real world." And in subjecting this awareness to constant discourse and displaying that discourse publicly, they offer the beginnings of a technique of repair.

Edge Play: Kinksters' Whips, Rabbis' Words, and the Dungeon of Study

If one can read rabbinic ritual impurity discourse as a conversation about managing risks that are unavoidable consequences of everyday life—that is, where risks are always present but in a low-grade manner that is not immediately central to the larger goal of social interaction—then the practice of text interpretation is where one might say the rabbis court significant risk head-on. It is significant, I argue, that the foundational activity around which the classical rabbinic community is formed and around which rabbis shape themselves as moral actors is one that is figured both as deeply risk laden and as desirable, pleasurable, and even seductive. Such a description also applies easily to organized BDSM and kink communities, for here, too, the community is formed and community members are shaped by a shared activity or set of activities that are physically, socially, and emotionally risky as well as being pleasurable and desirable for those who partake. In both cases, the community is formed around the risk activity as well as functioning as a system of risk management. In each case, furthermore, the activity is framed as somehow countercultural; it also accommodates a diversity of approaches and praxes under its aegis while simultaneously maintaining certain participatory norms designed to contain its inherent risks.

Perils of Peshaṭ and Dangers of Derash: Text Study as a Risk Activity

It is hardly a new observation that rabbinic texts, especially later ones such as the Bavli, saw the activity of Torah study as an activity that was simultaneously perilous and highly desirable. For example, as Jeffrey Rubenstein notes, the Bavli's argumentative rhetoric is explicitly violent: a sage who has been defeated in an argument may respond with predictions of his opponent's violent death or with threats against his opponent's family.[4] Importantly, the risks of this violent discourse are not merely rhetorical, for the distance between rhetoric and physical consequence in this universe is significantly collapsed: when rabbis speak and act in particular ways, things happen in the physical world. Rubenstein, for example, draws our attention to the story (discussed at the end of chapter 3) in B. Bava Metzia 84a, in which R. Yoḥanan's curse leads to Resh Laḳish's illness and death and in which the rabbis' subsequent prayers for mercy lead to R. Yoḥanan's own death. He also notes an episode in B. Yevamot 106a in which Abaye, miffed by Rav Papa's having made a clever point in his absence, searches out Rav Papa's parents and kills them with a single glance.[5] These texts assume, more often than not, that the rabbis have some kind of access to the divine, whether it be through their virtue, their knowledge, or the simple fact that they are working with the uniquely potent divine word, that allows them to affect material consequences in the world through their speech and ritual actions.

Along these lines, Torah's own words are also dangerous, especially to the sage who fails to respect their power. Per Jonathan Schofer, uninterpreted Written Torah especially may arouse sexual desire or incite anger, so one should engage it only through the safety lens of sagely interpretation.[6] But the acts of interpretation that counter the dangers of Written Torah hold their own perils, for they are vulnerable to falsification and doubt.[7] As Schofer puts it, in these texts "we see rabbinic reflection on the dangers of their own hermeneutic process."[8] Transgressions on a cosmic scale occur "through oral interpretation of the law in a rabbinic fashion."[9]

Yet it is not an option to avoid the carnage simply by exiting the field of play. Status in the Babylonian academy was, Rubenstein argues, intimately linked to the regular display of dialectical skill, and failure to participate for whatever reason could lead to a precipitous decline in status.[10] Furthermore, the fundamental social relationship for the Babylonian sage was the study-partner, or ḥavruta, with whom the sage could engage in particularly intense and extended dialectical warfare. The loss of this particular relationship was so devastating that, in some cases, "death would be preferable to such solitude."[11] Babylonian sages thus balanced carefully between competing dangers. They "depended on study partners for rigorous argumentation but simultaneously risked insulting their partners in the heat of debate," Rubenstein writes, adding: "A razor's edge seems to have separated intense argumentation—the prerequisite for rabbinic life—from verbal insults that could cause embarrassment and (social and metaphoric) death."[12] Sages' social status, identity, and psychosocial well-being were thus inextricably wrapped up in an activity that was violent, dangerous, all-consuming, and yet deeply life-giving.

Similarly, with the dangers of the text itself, risk is not the whole story. Torah and its interpretation are dangerous and tempting, but they are also life-giving and, if used correctly, function as a check against the same dangers that their injudicious use invites. Further, it is only through the activity of Torah study and what Schofer refers to as "willed subjection" to its curriculum that the sage is shaped into a virtuous actor. The texts imagine the human as having an evil *yetser*, or "inclination," that manifests itself as resistance to God's commands and a good yetser that is receptive to them; the activities of Torah study and performance of the commandments enable the good yetser to prevail. The sages in Avot D'Rabbi Natan compare Torah's process of combating the evil yetser and supporting the good yetser to a goad that keeps a draft animal in its furrow (A18:68), a blacksmith's fire (A16:64), and a warrior who conquers a city (A23:75, B33:72). What is notable about these metaphors in particular, from the many others that Schofer identifies in Avot D'Rabbi Natan, is that in these it is precisely an instrument of violence or danger that is responsible for guiding, shaping, or forcing the subject into the desired behavior or form. As Schofer writes regarding the goad metaphor in A18:68, "The teachings call upon the student to be docile and receptive, receiving the guidance and habituation that the Torah provides."[13] And, under this guidance, even the dangerous, self-centered, anarchic evil yetser can be disciplined and put to use.[14] That activity, in other words, that can tempt and kill can also shape and guide; in doing so, it can also bring other risky activities and inclinations under the yoke of discipline and put them to use.

One text that vividly displays the risky character, powerful desirability, and importance in shared identity formation of rabbinic text interpretation is the well-known Oven of Akhnai story, in Bavli Bava Metzia 59a–b. Often one of the first rabbinic texts to which a student of Judaism at the university level is introduced, this story is often deployed to demonstrate rabbinic irreverence or to make a point about the apparent arbitrariness of rabbinic hermeneutical method. Read in its immediate literary context, it is an object lesson about the dangers of verbally wronging or humiliating another. It can, however, also be productively read as an excursus on the manifold risks inherent in the activity of interpreting scripture in community.

In this passage—which is bracketed by excurses on honor, avoiding humiliation, and verbal wronging—the sages are debating whether a kind of clay oven, described in M. Kelim 5:10, remains ritually pure when it is cut into segments and sand is placed between them. This mishnah tells us that Rabbi Eliezer—a highly prominent and respected *tanna* known for his interpretive conservatism—declared such an oven pure, while the sages declared it susceptible to impurity. Such an oven, the Mishnah continues, is called the Oven of Akhnai, and at this point the Gemara takes over the story. We learn that the oven received its epithet because of the arguments with which the sages encircled it—and that during that confrontation, Rabbi Eliezer brings all the proof in the world. He should, on technical grounds, be winning this argument decisively right now. And yet the sages are unmoved:

> Why "*akhnai*" [a word whose root refers to both the act of encircling and to a snake]? R. Yehudah said that Shmuel said, because they surrounded it with arguments, like a snake, and declared it impure.[15]
> On that day, Rabbi Eliezer responded with all the answers in the world, but they did not accept them from him.

Rabbi Eliezer, we see, is at odds with the rest of the sages regarding the purity of the oven. And it is not as if he lacks sufficient support for his argument; indeed, he gives "all the answers in the world," but the sages do not accept them. Already, then, we see some evidence of how public debate carries inherent risk: one may be a venerated elder and expert with an abundance of data and rhetorical prowess at one's command and still be unable to sway one's community.

At this point, despite having solid logical grounds for his argument, Rabbi Eliezer plays a very risky game by continuing to oppose every other member of the academy. A more risk-averse figure might give up. Instead, Rabbi Eliezer becomes exasperated and ups the ante by invoking explicit divine power. He declares that if he's correct, the divine should prove it through a series of physically impossible events—to which the divine responds favorably!

> He said to them: if the halakhah is with me, let this carob tree prove it!
> The carob tree was uprooted from its place one hundred cubits—and some say, four hundred cubits.
> They said to him: we do not reason on the evidence of a carob tree!
> He shot back: if the halakhah is with me, let the stream prove it!
> The stream turned backward.
> They said to him: we do not reason on the evidence of a stream!

Rabbi Eliezer has exhausted his textual evidence and his rhetorical armory. He has technically done everything he should have to do to win, but his interlocutors remain unmoved, and so he has, more or less, thrown up his hands and cried, "Hashem, take the wheel!" In doing so, however, he has reminded the sages that they are not simply debating any text; rather, they are talking about divine language. This distinction has tangible consequences, and Rabbi Eliezer clearly has enough standing with the divine realm to invoke these supernatural effects in support of his position. The sages, however, are unwilling to suspend the community's normal rules of play, even in the face of clearly abnormal circumstances.

In the next set of exchanges, the sages demonstrate an awareness of these abnormal circumstances—but they do so in a way that reasserts the normal rules of play by treating the divine as yet another debater. Rabbi Eliezer declares that if he's correct, the walls of the very building should incline; Rabbi Yehoshua rebukes the divine for meddling in the business of the sages, and in response to these equally compelling claims, the walls remain indecisive:

> [R. Eliezer] retorted: if the halakhah is with me, let the walls of the bet midrash prove it! The walls of the bet midrash leaned and began to fall.
> R. Yehoshua scolded [the walls] and said to them, "If sages are contending with each other regarding halakhah, what business have you?!"
> [The walls] did not fall on account of R. Yehoshua's honor, but they did not straighten on account of R. Eliezer's honor. They still stand inclined.

R. Eliezer, who seems to have reached the end of his tether here, retorts with the baldest appeal to divine power yet: if, he cries, he's correct, let it be proven directly from the source! Heaven remains with him, and a divine voice supports him directly. Rabbi Yehoshua, however, in an act that is perhaps the dictionary definition of chutzpah, tells the divine voice to mind its own business, and he does so by quoting scripture:

> [R. Eliezer] then retorted: if the halakhah is with me, let it be proven from Heaven!
>
> A *bat ḳol* [divine voice] emerged and said, "why are you at it with R. Eliezer, given that the halakhah is with him in every place?"
>
> R. Yehoshua stood on his feet and said, "it is not in Heaven!" (Deut. 30:12)
>
> What is the relevance of "it is not in Heaven?"
>
> R. Yirmiyah said: since the Torah was already given at Mt. Sinai, we pay no mind to a bat ḳol, as You already wrote at Mt. Sinai in the Torah, "after a majority to incline." (Ex. 23:2)

It's worth noting here that if we look at the scripture Rabbi Yehoshua's quoting, he comes across as even more audacious. The passage, from Deuteronomy 30:11–12—"Surely, this instruction which I enjoin upon you this day is not too baffling for you, nor is it beyond reach. It is not in the heavens, that you should say, 'Who among us can go up to the heavens and get it for us and impart it to us, that we may observe it?'"—is from the Song of Moses, and it is part of a sequence in which Moses is, not to put too fine a point on it, informing the entire people Israel that they are stubborn, perfidious blockheads. Quite a passage to quote at a voice from God, indeed.

Rabbi Yehoshua, then, is playing a game of risk at the highest level. His opponent's argument has literally been affirmed by a voice from above, the voice of an entity that has just demonstrated its power to move trees, incline walls, and make streams flow backward—and Rabbi Yehoshua has just, in effect, mouthed off to it and done so by quoting its own words. This is, however, an entity that has indicated its willingness, at least on some level, to play R. Yehoshua's game: the walls remain only partly inclined in deference to R. Yehoshua's act of negotiation. The inclined synagogue walls stand as a physical testimony to a metaphysical stalemate, as well as to the power of even mere mortals' play with divine words. And the potential rewards of Rabbi Yehoshua's gambit are made even clearer by Eliyahu the prophet's subsequent report: God has taken note of God's subjects' play and is both impressed and amused.

> R. Natan encountered Eliyahu the prophet, and said to him: What did the Holy One, Blessed be God, do at that time?
>   He said to him: God smiled, and said, "My children have defeated Me, My children have defeated Me."

Yet if the extreme risks Rabbi Yehoshua and the sages take by standing against a divinely backed Rabbi Eliezer are on one level rewarded by explicit divine recognition and approval of their cleverness and boldness, the dangers—metaphysical, moral, and social—of their take-no-prisoners approach are also extreme. In the aftermath of the debate over the oven, the improbably defeated Rabbi Eliezer is excommunicated and his rulings rendered invalid—the ultimate act of public shaming: "[The sages] said: on that day they brought out all the pure things that R. Eliezer had declared pure, and burned them in a fire, and they voted on him and shunned him." We see in this development the social aspect of the risks and rewards of the rabbinic community. In losing his place among the sages and his communally recognized authority, Rabbi Eliezer has lost nearly everything in the social world that sustains him and that constitutes his identity. He is humiliated, hurt, and socially ruined. He has given everything to a community that, in the end, has the power to humiliate even such a powerful figure as himself. Even the great Rabbi Eliezer is not immune to communal violence.

Rabbi Eliezer is not, however, divinely abandoned, and in this way the community that was able to hurt him remains deeply vulnerable to the consequences of their own extreme actions. Rabbi Akiva, at least, seems aware enough of the stakes of this game to enact some risk-management strategies:

> [The sages] said: who will go and inform him?
>   R. Akiva said to them: I will go, lest an unfit person should go and inform him and he should thereby destroy the entire world.
>   What did Rabbi Akiva do? He wore black and draped himself in black, and sat before [R. Eliezer] at a distance of four *amot*.[16]
>   R. Eliezer said to him: Akiva, what [is different] about today than other days?
>   He said to him: My teacher, it seems to me that our colleagues are keeping aloof from you.
>   Thereupon R. Eliezer tore his clothes and cast off his shoes, and he slipped [from his chair] and sat upon the ground. His eyes dripped tears, and so the

world was stricken: one third of its olives, and one third of its wheat, and one third of its barley. And some say, even the dough spoiled in a woman's hands.

[The sages] taught: there was great calamity on that day, for any place upon which R. Eliezer set his eyes was burned.

Despite Rabbi Aḳiva's attempts at harm reduction, the consequences of shaming Rabbi Eliezer prove dire. The raw power of his pain and sorrow causes crops to fail and food to spoil, and the ground is burned wherever he fixes his (weeping) gaze. In fact, first the created world and then heaven itself respond so strongly and precisely to Rabbi Eliezer's wounding that they specifically target Raban Gamaliel, the *naśi*, that is, the leader of the rabbinic assembly that excommunicated Rabbi Eliezer. First, a rogue wave threatens to inundate a ship on which Raban Gamaliel is traveling, but he is able to reason with the wave and talk it down:

And even Raban Gamaliel was coming on a boat, and a crushing swell stood over him, threatening to drown him.

He said: it seems to me that this can only be on account of R. Eliezer ben Hyrcanus.

He stood on his feet and said: Master of the Universe, it is revealed and known before you that I acted neither for my own honor, nor did I act for the honor of my father's house. Rather, it was for Your honor, so that disputes would not multiply in Israel.

The sea calmed its raging.

When it comes to the consequences of Rabbi Eliezer's prayers, however, Raban Gamaliel is not so lucky:

Ima Shalom, the wife of Rabbi Eliezer, was the sister of Raban Gamaliel. Thenceforward, she would not allow R. Eliezer to fall on his face [in order to recite the Taḥanun prayer of entreaty and supplication].

A certain day was around the New Moon, and she confused a full [month] with a diminished one [thereby assuming it was Rosh Ḥodesh, when one does not recite Taḥanun] Some say: a beggar came and stood at the door, and she brought out bread to him.

She found him having fallen on his face [in prayer].

She said to him: Get up. You have killed my brother.

Meanwhile, the cry of a shofar came out from the house of Raban Gamaliel, [announcing] that he had died.

He said to her: How did you know?

She said to him: I received this from the house of my father's father: all gates are locked, save for the gates of verbal wronging.

Notably, Rabbi Eliezer does not seem to have control over any of these retributive phenomena. It is as though his grief over his excommunication is a force unto itself, which then triggers first abnormal phenomena in the created world and then specific responses from the divine. It is also notable here that it is Rabbi Eliezer's wife—by definition an outsider to the rabbinic community—who recognizes the specific danger that comes of Rabbi Eliezer's prayers and is able to cite a received chain of transmission from which she learned this.

The cosmic response to rabbinic edge play gone out of control in this story is rather extreme even by Talmudic standards. Yet the story aptly demonstrates several features of the series of risks and rewards inherent to the rabbis' communal interpretive practices. The potential for social fracturing and personal loss of social standing among an already small and marginalized community highlights the high stakes of that community's valuation of pitched, intense, and often vicious disputation as the central, affinity-generating, identity-forming activity upon which it is built. The risk is heightened by the subject matter of this disputation play: the story reminds us that the rabbis are fighting over the words of God, which are powerful and volatile things in their own right; as such, this play has potential physical, social, and metaphysical consequences. And Rabbi Eliezer's exasperated invocation of direct divine power adds yet another level of cosmic danger to the play.

All the same, the discourse is clearly well aware of its multiply risky character. Indeed, the inclusion of this extreme story, especially coming, as it does, in the context of a longer discussion about the harms of verbal wronging and humiliation, may be read itself as a risk-management practice. Interpersonal virtues, including virtues of careful speech and preserving the dignity of one's peers, are important, the Gemara seems to say. This is doubly true for the risky communal practices of interpretation and disputation of sacred text that define the sagely self and form the rabbinic community, and so there are best practices for this kind of discourse. And in case you doubted the importance of scrupulous attention to and cultivation of these best practices, the Gemara adds, let us demonstrate for you the full stakes of the game you are playing. Now, perhaps, you understand why such care might be called for?

Between the Dungeon and the Bet Midrash: Communal Responses to Risk

In contrast with the activity of rabbinic text interpretation, it is hardly necessary to establish BDSM practice as a risk activity. BDSM scenes by definition involve playing with potentially painful or dangerous situations, instruments, sensations, and power dynamics; as one of the anthropologist Staci Newmahr's informants in *Playing on the Edge: Sadomasochism, Risk, and Intimacy* puts it, "Many SM participants are putting themselves into situations in which they truly could be powerless."[17] BDSM play may involve varying degrees of bondage, flogging, caning, and even knife play and breath play. There is little question that BDSM is risky; there is also little question that it is often precisely its risky character that is responsible for its appeal.

As the bet midrash is a community formed around the practice of discursive text interpretation, I argue that organized BDSM groups are also communities that are organized around a risk activity, that said risk activity is critical to its members' identity formation, and that communities' norms serve to shape and discipline their members in particular ways. Organized BDSM communities are communities of moral formation, and BDSM practice is a form of habitus. Further, I argue that, because much of the most prominent risk-management strategy found in organized BDSM is based in discourse and negotiation, there is more of an overlap of technique between BDSM practitioners and the rabbis than one might expect. Risk, in both cases, is sought out and celebrated; in both cases it is also controlled largely through discussion. Finally, I argue, the formative affinities of organized BDSM communities accommodate and even seek to affirm sociosexual diversity; as such, they offer resources for a model of community formation that, rather than flattening or eliding diversity, depends on it for its flourishing.

Acknowledgment of the risky character of BDSM is built explicitly into its foundational shared language. Two terms denote two related but distinct visions of what might be called a general ethical foundation for BDSM culture writ large: "Safe, Sane, and Consensual" (SSC) and "risk-aware consensual kink" (RACK). The former was coined in 1983 in a "statement of identity and purpose" for New York's Gay Male S/M Activists, as a way of distinguishing their practices from sexual and physical abuse. The latter is attributed to Gary Switch, who in 1999 wrote that he found the term *sane* vague and *safe* misleading, arguing that "mountain climbers don't call their sport safe, for the simple reason that it isn't; risk is an essential part of the thrill. They handle it by identifying and minimizing the risk through study, training, technique, and practice."[18] In either case, however, consent remains the linchpin of BDSM ethics and culture. Consent is meant to be the definitive boundary between BDSM and abuse, even if both may involve inflicting physical or psychological injury. In practice, the term *consent* covers not only any given agreement to an activity but includes participants' state of mind and the content and formal structure of their ongoing negotiation of what will and will not occur for the duration of BDSM activity.[19]

To participate in organized BDSM and manage this acknowledged risk, one must devote a great deal of time to learning a particular set of technical and social skills. "Learning to play," writes Newmahr, "is an integral part of becoming a sadomasochist, shaping motivations and forming identities in the process."[20] These practices of identity formation serve to positively distinguish BDSM practitioners from other people; Weiss relates that one of her informants referred to BDSM as "graduate school sex," adding that "it is this kind of educational mastery that differentiates—as Malc, a white, heterosexual, mostly dominant in his late thirties put it—'people who are identified as BDSM practitioners and people who just do rough sex.'"[21] To become a true practitioner, one who is fully integrated in a BDSM community, occurs through "participation in a social, sexual, and educational community that teaches techniques of the self alongside rope bondage and flogging skills."[22] So BDSM practice is play, but it is play that constructs and shapes identities and roles throughout participants' lives. Players' identities as dominant, submissive, or switch, for example, are adopted within play space but remain significant well outside of particular scenes.

Here, then, risk, in Weiss's words, is "productive; building and mastering BDSM skills produce new subjects in relation to an evaluative community. The community evaluates one's education, trustworthiness, experience, and skill."[23] Inhabiting and performing one's cultivated skills and chosen labels are critical components of successful social intercourse within the BDSM community, since "networking for play [is] an important component of the social scene. Misleading labels can be at the root of unproductive flirting, messy or unclear scene negotiations, and, ultimately bad scenes. Bad scenes, in turn, have the potential to breed bad reputations, [and] bad reputations [can] be extremely detrimental to a person who wants to engage in SM play."[24] The identities players cultivate—both their labels and their reputations as safe and skilled players and, eventually, educators—both reinforce the community's formative affinities and contribute to players' senses of self and their mastery of their experiences and their responses to them. These players, Newmahr argues, "are not [donning] and stripping these identities as one might change costumes. Rather they are actively constructing experiences in which they can *feel* relatively powerful or powerless, not through their own performances, in the theatrical sense, but through the cooperative performances, in the Goffmanian sense, of all community members."[25]

As with the rabbinic community, mastery of the community's constitutive skills and of the self is important both for its own sake and for the sake of managing the risk activities around which that community is formed. Newmahr notes that "even apart from participants' general desires to avoid sustenance and infliction of unintended injury themselves, the community as a whole shares responsibility for recruitment, education, and supervision of SM play. SM is taught, supervised, policed, and regulated in multiple ways."[26] While Newmahr de-emphasizes specific risk management here, it is nevertheless noteworthy that she frames education in particular—much of which is devoted to cultivating skills that are essential to managing and reducing the native risks of BDSM practice—as a collective responsibility. The technical skills that new BDSM players must cultivate and experienced players must hone and maintain help mitigate risks of permanent injury and infection; additionally, the social performance of skill and competence helps cultivate an atmosphere in which players feel willing to relax, trust partners, and proceed calmly through the scene.

Hermeneutic competency is just as critical for risk management as technical skill. Because, as Newmahr notes, "direct communication [within a scene] threatens power performances and handicaps the accomplishment of 'pushing limits,' [tops must learn] to decode communication strategies in play and to recognize signals that the bottom may or may not intend to send. . . . Tops must often decode ambiguous, conflicting, or barely visible signals in order to avoid causing real damage to play partners."[27] Bottoms, too, must learn particular skills and techniques of the self, although, as Newmahr notes, "the processes are less obvious" since tops usually hold direct responsibility for safety and for the proper use of the techniques and apparatus used on the bottom.[28] Nevertheless, bottoms are formed in both self-facing and other-facing ways: they learn to "give themselves 'permission' to recognize and understand their likes, dislikes and limits, as well as how to communicate those things in scene and out of scene," to "evaluate their limits—'hard' limits that should be left alone, or 'soft' limits that may be pushed by the top," "criteria for playing safely, such as how to choose a play partner wisely and disclose concerns, issues, and health problems," and how to "process, navigate, and negotiate pain or unpleasant sensation."[29]

Regardless of a player's chosen labels, nearly all BDSM scenes should begin with negotiation—often rather formal—which precedes the acting out of the scene and continues in some form throughout. This can be as formalized as a checklist, or it may take the shape of looser verbal negotiation; regardless, it will address questions like who will participate, where the scene will occur and how long it will last, what activities will definitely be included and what activities are off-limits, players' emotional and physical limits or triggers, whether any marks may be left on the body, and safe words.[30] In particular, safe words (or a nonverbal equivalent, like a series of hand squeezes, for situations in which a player is gagged or otherwise unable to speak) are an important discursive and interpretive technique for keeping the conversation about consent and limits open throughout the scene. It is considered best practice to have a two-stage safe signal, where a "softer" version communicates "pause" or "take it easy" and a harder version halts all play temporarily or permanently.

The centrality of formal negotiation as a fundamental risk-management strategy is one of the most notable features of organized BDSM communities. In this way, as with the rabbis, the kink community's "best practices" for risk management are *discursive* best practices—they are practices that ask members to shape themselves in particular moral directions by way of disciplining their words according to specific frameworks, and which depend on cultivating a high level of hermeneutic competency. These frameworks are not rigid and uniformity inducing; just as the pitched debate the rabbinic community thrives on is not possible without the existence of different opinions and different schools or traditions of interpretive debate, so too, the structure of negotiation expected in BDSM play allows for considerable variation. For example, Karen Johanns, in an essay in the 1988 *Lesbian S/M Safety Manual*, suggests ways that pre-negotiation can be worked into the setting of the scene itself—negotiations can take the form of a sex survey administered by a researcher, for example, or a disciplinary interview in a school setting.[31] Such negotiation structures, as Weiss argues, ask players to "negotiate their own relationship to these rules to define safety and risk for themselves."[32]

Indeed, for all that organized BDSM is a community that tenders formal rules of interaction and asks its members to discipline and shape themselves in specific, community-directed ways, it is also a community that is formed precisely around difference, as a place where one of the foundational and community-forming affinities is that of sexual divergence. It therefore, at least to some extent, necessarily cultivates a form of diverse interdependence among its members. As such, it has the potential, at least prima facie, to answer Rey Chow's question about whether "sexual difference [could] ever be reconciled with community" in the affirmative.[33] Here, we see a community whose raison d'être is to provide a space for a range of sociosexual misfits and a social support network in which they can express and discuss sexualities that are suppressed or discouraged by broader social hegemonies. And, indeed, there are ways in which the sexually marginal identities that organized BDSM affirms are linked to other socially marginal identities as well. Kathy Sisson tracks the emergence of specific gay and lesbian BDSM communities in the 1940s and 1970s, the latter perhaps not coincidentally emerging at the height of a significant period in the gay liberation movement.[34] The HIV/ AIDS epidemic also sparked a period of considerable political development for the BDSM community.[35] And Newmahr notes that many of her informants shared other socially marginal interests and identities: many were fat, socially awkward, or had "geeky" interests; some were mentally ill, and many had experienced some kind of familial trauma growing up.[36] The physical and social bodies of BDSMers, then, are deviant in multiple ways. But they are not, as dominant sexual hierarchies would have it, undisciplined—indeed, as I have shown, these bodies are highly disciplined. The innovation of the BDSM community is to create a context for such communal discipline that, at its best, can *highlight* diversity rather than flattening it.

Models for Moral Community

The bet midrash as we see it described in classical texts is, like organized BDSM communities, a community based on shared participation in a strongly desired risk activity, participation that, in turn, is significantly constitutive of participants' identities. Each community cultivates disciplines among its participants that further shape those participants' identities and behaviors in specific and desirable directions. These similarities between the two spaces also point toward ways in which both communities can model sexual and more broadly social virtues. In particular, I argue, these communities offer models for a robust communal ethic in which difference, idiosyncrasy, and individual needs and preferences are not ironed out or elided but rather actively contribute to communal flourishing and are developed as virtues in their own right.

The first way in which what I shall call *risk-conditioned communities* model social virtues is in their broad assumption that disciplines practiced in and for a very specific social context are in fact valuable and applicable outside that context. This is more obvious in the rabbinic context, in which disciplines of study and prayer are explicitly linked to broader moral formation.[37] It is, however, also the case for BDSM players: several of Newmahr's subjects, for example, described feeling outcast or otherwise socially marginal. The community they find in BDSM spaces affords them a sense of belonging, and the specific skills they cultivate give them accomplishments in which they can take real pride, pride that in turn translates to a greater sense of social confidence and self-esteem.[38]

Second, risk-conditioned communities also model the development of broader virtues through the practice of specific technical and social skills. In particular, the two risk-conditioned communities I treat here foster the development of hermeneutic competency as a skill of both technical and moral import and as a critical component of the specific sorts of wise risk management their central activities clearly require. Organized BDSM places extraordinary value on the ability to negotiate with a partner and to interpret that partner's communication—both verbal and nonverbal—to determine how and whether to proceed in a given encounter. Such hermeneutic care requires deep social attentiveness and concern for an interlocutor's well-being. The importance of such is made sharply clear in an obviously risk-laden context like BDSM, but exactly the same skills are also critical tools for being a good social actor more generally.

In particular, the ways consent functions within such risk-conditioned communities are instructive well beyond their specific contexts. One of the most fundamental critiques of what can often be a simplistic reliance on consent within much contemporary sex-positive culture is that it is basically individualistic, placing outsized responsibility on single actors, failing to account for the ways in which the choice to consent to a given act in a given circumstance is conditioned both directly and indirectly by the social structures one inhabits, and stymying the construction and enforcement of broader communal norms. In the highly ritualized play of organized BDSM, however, consent is not an act that a single agent performs once. It is a discursive framework, a social scaffold upon which community members structure ongoing interactions with one another. Consent in this context has recognizable formal markers: scenes are pre-negotiated, and frameworks for ongoing negotiation and communication of consent or its withdrawal (for example, a safe word progression of "green, yellow, red" in which green means "keep going," yellow means "pause" or "slow down," and red means "stop everything right now") are put into place. The structures are modifiable enough to account for variation among practitioners and the particulars of scenes (e.g., allowing for nonverbal safe word structures in situations where one or more players may be gagged), but there is nevertheless community oversight of and participation in their development, maintenance, and general recognizability.

Participating in such formalized-yet-flexible structures of negotiation on a regular basis can shape moral actors to be attentive to a range of modes of communication (hermeneutic competency) throughout their social lives. It can likewise shape practitioners to be proactive about attending to people's needs, desires, and well-being, instead of assuming that because others have not explicitly discussed a course of action that they are adequately comfortable with it.

Hermeneutic competency is likewise a basic requirement for participation in rabbinic discourse, and, as episodes like the tanur shel akhnai make clear, the risks that participants engage are great enough that sometimes even the hermeneutic competency of masters is insufficient to manage it fully. Like the discourse of negotiated and ongoing consent in BDSM, the hermeneutic discourse of the bet midrash is practiced according to communally recognized formal patterns, even as it admits sometimes significant variation within those patterns. Rabbinic discourse also offers a model of how to do this kind of practice with the awareness that one's interpretive and communicative choices, acts, and insights are conditioned by actors and structures outside of oneself. Whether these are the scholarly tradition from which one learns one's skills (explicitly marked when rabbis speak in the name of so-and-so or even a chain of so-and-sos), the political context of occupation and subjection at the hands of the Roman empire, the destruction of the temple and the transition from temple-based to text-based practice, or the scriptural and divine source material that everyone works with (explicitly marked throughout the tanur shel akhnai episode), the rabbis are all too clear that they do not act in a vacuum. Such explicit awareness and, indeed, building that awareness into the formal structure of the community's hermeneutic praxis could potentially begin to address the (valid) critique that consent culture often elides these influences.

Finally and, to my mind, most critically, both of the risk-conditioned communities I treat here promote and cultivate specific shared virtues and skills without eliminating difference. This is a matter of particular import for sexual ethics because, as I have noted at multiple points, the field of religious sexual ethics as a whole has had a frustrating tendency to flatten questions of sexual practice into a shallow discourse of individual versus community, one in which variations in sexual behaviors or preferences become representative of a caricatured individualism and in which true participation in community requires the disciplined suppression of most such variation. In organized BDSM, however, diverse interdependence is central. Organized BDSM demonstrates that it is more than possible for a community to encourage the development of particular common virtues and to set limits on the universe of allowable practice while still allowing for and indeed encouraging a wide array of practices and preferences within that universe. Such a model is also present, in a different way, in the bet midrash: here, too, common disciplines of piety, reading practice, and hermeneutical skill are enforced; at the same time, the universe of legitimate rabbinic interpretive practice accommodates and indeed thrives on the interplay and conflict among multiple distinct approaches to interpretation, law, ethics, and theology. What is, however, secondary and limited in the bet midrash is a foundational premise in the BDSM dungeon.

As I am about to discuss in the next section, just because sexual diversity (and by extension, diversity in general) is a foundational affinity in organized BDSM practice does not mean that the lived realities of BDSM always live up to that ideal. As Weiss's work convincingly shows, despite its rhetorics of refuge and separation from and transgression of the pernicious hierarchies of broader social hegemonies, it is in fact intimately connected to and therefore dependent on and reproductive of those very same hierarchies. Ironically, its rhetorics of separateness may, Weiss suggests, be counterproductive to its stated transgressive aims, and for this, as we shall see, the rabbis may offer a corrective. But in founding a community on an ideal of diversity and difference and, indeed, of productive social transgression, organized BDSM has a corrective for us all.

Power Play: Escapism and Appropriation, or, When Have the Romans Ever Played with Us?

Doing a practice, text, or community empirical justice means paying attention to the range ways it functions in the real world, for the people actually engaged with it. This means, among other things, attending to and acknowledging the things it does well. In the previous section, I discussed ways that BDSM communities and the bet midrash as we see it portrayed in rabbinic literature model virtuous ways of accommodating and, indeed, affirming diverse practices and predilections around a risky social activity within a cohesive community. Doing a subject empirical justice, however, also means attending to and acknowledging the ways it is problematic. As I noted in chapter 1, a given rabbinic text may offer a positive model for a contemporary problem—that is, it may offer a way of thinking about or dealing with the problem that improves in some way on what is already being done. But it may also offer a negative model—that is, it may demonstrate poor reasoning or practice in a way that elucidates similarly poor reasoning or practice in the contemporary situation or warns against similar poor practice if current trends continue unchecked. Further, positive and negative models can and often do coexist within a single case study.

Thus, here, rabbinic accommodation of diverse practices within a community organized around a risky practice parallels similar features of BDSM communities and offers a helpful model for managing risk and affirming diversity within communities—a model, furthermore, that does not rely on classic individualist "rights" language. At the same time, BDSM communities can reproduce deeply troubling power dynamics; further, due to communities' narratives of their own disempowerment given their status as sexual minorities, these dynamics may well go unexamined. Here, I argue, rabbinic discourse provides both a negative example that serves to elucidate aspects of how these power dynamics are reproduced and a positive example that serves to demonstrate at least one potential path to greater self-awareness. As Beth Berkowitz demonstrates in *Execution and Invention: Death Penalty Discourse in Early Rabbinic and Christian Cultures*, the rabbis, in the ways they imagined rituals of execution, appropriated and reproduced features and symbols of Roman imperial power, positioning themselves not only in opposition to the authority of the Roman empire but as authorities above their fellow Jews. At the same time, however, Berkowitz shows that there is a self-awareness and even a certain ironic "wink" in this appropriation: the rabbis, in some important ways, know exactly what they are doing. They know they are in dialogue with Rome and—ironically, since it is likely that the rituals of execution they imagine were never carried out—do not assume that their "execution play," as it were, exists in a universe separate from the realities of oppression and empire.

Circuits of Sexuality: Kink, Class, and Capital

The anthropologist Margot Weiss, in *Techniques of Pleasure: BDSM and the Circuits of Sexuality*, observes that organized BDSM play, despite its escapist rhetoric, often reproduces many of the power dynamics of its capitalist and white supremacist context. This is because, first of all, "SM functions as a space of belonging, a *community* with all of the vexed striving toward an ultimately failed inclusion that this term conveys."[39] Organized BDSM is a community in the basic Sandelian sense I discussed in chapter 2: it is "a social group organized around some sort of affinity or affinities that its members understand as somehow significantly constitutive of their individual and collective identities and which is structured in a way that promotes the further development of those characteristics that are conducive to maintaining affinity." And, as I discussed in the previous section, organized BDSM avoids, at least on some level, the all-too-pervasive failure of communities to accommodate and affirm internal difference and diversity, especially where gender and sexuality are concerned; rather, such diversity seems built into the very identity-forming affinity that creates the community to begin with.

However, Weiss, following Miranda Joseph, argues that community, specifically modern and postmodern community, "does not exist outside of the relations of production, forms of leisure and labor, spatial geography, and other configurations of capitalism that it both depends on and reproduces. *Indeed, it is precisely because this community is so bound to social and economic relations that it functions as a community.*"[40] The current generation of pansexual BDSM players connect via electronic media, and they reinforce and continually shape their shared identity through the cultivation of physical, social, and economic techniques. And, notably, many of these techniques require significant outlays of economically significant resources: time, attention, and money.

Indeed, at least according to some of Weiss's informants, there is a direct relationship between economic outlay and status within the community: for example, "the inability to buy the latest or best toy relegates one to a second-tier belonging in the community."[41] Similarly, play parties often have door fees that may prove inaccessible. While one can exchange one's volunteer labor on behalf of the party for free entry, Weiss's informants describe this labor as tiring, logistically tricky, and often humiliating. Door fees thus function as another way "that the community creates tiers of classed belonging."[42] Ultimately, Weiss argues, "belonging to the SM community and being a recognized practitioner is bound to income: the assumption that one has the money to play."[43]

Class is not the only system that BDSM communities can reify. Gender, race, ethnicity, able-bodiedness, and, ironically enough, sexuality are all categories with which organized BDSM has complex, often problematic, and often un- or underacknowledged relationships. Central to classical radical feminist condemnation of BDSM is the claim that any practice that eroticizes pain, objectification, and unequal power dynamics necessarily is produced by and reproduces these pernicious dynamics in society writ large.[44] Pro-BDSM voices may counter that, in one way or another, the spaces in which BDSM occurs are somehow distinct from the spaces in which "genuine" oppression does: either claiming that sex is "primarily a private issue, divorced from political considerations," or making the more nuanced argument that, because BDSM occurs within a context of self-aware performance and play, the replication of pernicious dynamics happens with an ironic and subversive wink.[45] Especially since players are allowed to choose their roles in the scene regardless of their "real-world" identities, this ironic reenactment allows players to manipulate, mock, transgress, and subvert those roles.[46] Alternatively, pro-BDSM voices argue that BDSM subverts forces of heteronormativity through its self-consciously performative character, insisting on taking deliberately deviant sexuality outside of its appointed private sphere.[47] In either case, the argument goes, the fundamentally queer (in the broad sense) world of BDSM knows what problematic sexual, gender, and racial hierarchies are, and by virtue of performatively engaging those hierarchies in queer spaces or from queer standpoints, it can create a community in which those dynamics are less likely to be reproduced.

Yet the demographic realities of organized BDSM practice, at least where Weiss's informants are concerned, prove somewhat resistant to this subversion. Among Weiss's contemporary pansexual BDSM practitioners, despite rhetoric celebrating the opportunity to reverse entrenched roles, "the majority of heterosexual couples were male dominant/female submissive."[48] Sexism and racism, for Weiss's informants, are live problems in the BDSM scene: "Women of all SM orientations reported that some men assume they must be submissive.... These assumptions are also racialized; [Weiss's informant] Bonne explained: '[As an Asian American,] I get a lot of men talking to me as if I'm supposed to be quiet and submissive.'"[49] These realities, as well as the above-discussed ways in which BDSM practice is enmeshed in and reproduces classed and economic hierarchies, point toward a more complicated relationship between BDSM practice and the real-life power dynamics it reenacts and, indeed, must draw on to generate its erotic power. For, as both Weiss and Newmahr demonstrate, BDSM practice is not just ironic performance: it is also a community-generated and generating cultivation of the self in specific directions. So while the self-awareness of this continued practice does create an opportunity to subvert the scripts members must work with, at the same time, "the need to stage a culturally recognizable performance relies on these original [scripts]," and in this, the cultural texts players work with both consciously and unconsciously exert influence on players even as players exert influence on the scripts. As Weiss puts it, "Mimetic performance produces subject who embody and cultivate social norms, even more than they subvert or consolidate them, at the same time that it produces the 'regulatory ideal' of the norms themselves."[50] Yet, according to Weiss, players often hold the ways in which they reproduce the scripts they want to subvert at arm's length by maintaining the narrative that BDSM is "mere" play: "It is only the fantasized break from the real of power—the scene as a safe space— that enables practitioners, and theorists, to imagine that in-scene gender is *only* a copy or a performance, that it has no social effects."[51]

So to play with these structures is a risk, and yet it is a risk that is impossible not to undertake. This, perhaps, is particularly obvious regarding BDSM, which by definition is risk conditioned. Yet Weiss's account shows that the political risks of such play can be insidious, as players use the screen of play to insulate themselves against the full implications of the real social texts they perform. BDSM is not the simple reproduction of pernicious social dynamics. But neither is it indemnified against them. Rather, it participates in them in complex ways, some transgressive, subversive, and revolutionary and others collaborative and supportive. Yet ironically, for a community whose identity-forming affinity is precisely playing with and embodying risky scripts, Weiss's subjects often fail to take seriously the ways play as ritual and script as text are real, socially enmeshed, and politically potent. I turn now to a group of players—the rabbis of the tannaitic period—who, for all that they are in many ways far less diverse and socially progressive than Weiss's pansexual BDSM communities, understand the real power of ritual and text all too well.

Circuits of Ritual: Exegesis, Execution, and Empire

Weiss convincingly shows that the relationship between organized BDSM and the systems it seeks to resist is a complicated one that reproduces and is intertwined with precisely those systems in intricate ways. Beth Berkowitz observes a similar phenomenon in the rabbis' relationship to Roman power through their own rituals of execution. Using theoretical resources from Foucault and from the postcolonial theorists Homi Bhabha and James Scott, Berkowitz reads rabbinic discourses of execution as, in Scott's words, a "hidden transcript" that evinces "the appropriation and resistance that is often embedded within postures of submission."[52] The execution rituals described in tannaitic texts, Berkowitz argues, are shaped "both to resemble Roman executions but also to be their opposite." Yet, she adds, "in the course of these reversals, the Rabbis allow themselves to come dangerously close to looking very much like the authority they eschew."[53] Further, Berkowitz shows, in systematizing and ritualizing the steps of a properly orchestrated execution—regardless of whether such would ever have been carried out, since the actual legal and political authority of the tannaim in their own historical context is in serious question—the rabbis consolidated their own authority within their own textual world, therefore erecting intracommunal hierarchies that they dominated even as they also expressed resistance to Roman hierarchy from a position of defiant if complex subalternity.

Berkowitz reads M. Sanhedrin 7:3, which describes execution by beheading—one of four permitted methods of execution, the others being stoning, burning, and strangulation—as a paradigm text for the rabbis' ironic mimicry of Roman power structures. That this text centers on beheading is not accidental, as it most closely resembles Roman methods. Here, the sages and Rabbi Judah dispute which way of carrying out a beheading is more "disgraceful" (niṿul). The sages argue that beheading is to be done with a sword, "in the manner that the kingdom does it." Rabbi Judah, however, disagrees:

> The mitzvah concerning decapitation: they would cut off his head with a sword, in the way that the kingdom does it.
> R. Yehudah said: that is disgraceful. Rather, they should rest his head on a block and chop it with a hatchet.
> [The sages] said to him: there is no death more disgraceful than this.

Execution as the sages recommend, Rabbi Judah argues, is a disgrace, so much so that he prefers "the tools of the butcher."[54] The sages respond that Rabbi Judah's method is even more disgraceful than the method he condemns.

While the language of this mishnah is elliptical and vague, what is at issue here—keeping in mind that the condemned is assumed to be a fellow Jew— is maintaining bodily and social dignity and how much the sociopolitical resonances of the method of execution matter to that end. This rests on the meanings of two terms in this mishnah: niṿul, or "disgrace," and the reference to decapitation by sword as k'derekh she'ha'malkhut ośah, "in the manner that the kingdom does it." Both terms, while obscure on their own, are elucidated through lexical comparison. As Berkowitz explains, in other tannaitic contexts, niṿul has to do with the degradation of the body, especially in sexualized ways: in several instances it refers to both women and men who lose or otherwise lack sexual appeal, whether through age, poverty, or, for men, congenital emasculation.[55] And *k' derekh she'ha'malkhut ośah*, when referring to execution and especially to the sword as it does here, has strong associations with Roman imperial might: the only other tannaitic use of the verbatim phrase also refers to Roman execution methods, and the motif of the sword in other tannaitic sources consistently symbolizes non-Jewish capital authority, especially Roman authority.[56]

The sages seem to be arguing that the Roman style of decapitation best preserves the bodily and sexual dignity of the Jewish condemned, whereas Rabbi Judah argues that, material optics (the resemblance to butchery) aside, the greatest indignity is to adopt Roman practices. Berkowitz notes that "under the Roman penal system, decapitation was a relatively honorable way to die, reserved generally for the upper-class condemned."[57] So, reading the sages' discourse as a "hidden transcript," one can see them as subversively appropriating the method of execution (execution itself being a power reserved for Rome) that the conquerors used for their most honored subjects to uplift even the lowliest—the condemned—of conquered (and thereby feminized) subjects to the status of a patrician. As Berkowitz writes, "The sages adapt the form of Roman execution [in] an effort to adapt the language of power and, in so doing, to challenge it."[58]

Rabbi Judah, however, is claiming that the sages, in appropriating Roman techniques of capital authority, do far worse than mere physical and social degradation. This is drawn out further, in modified form, in t. Sanhedrin 9:11, the parallel tosefta to this mishnah, which preserves Rabbi Judah's retort to the sages' admonition that there is no execution more disgraceful than that done by ax on the chopping block:[59] "He said to them: of course there is no death more disgraceful than this; rather, this is because, as it is stated, 'nor shall you follow their laws'" (Lev. 18:3). In doing so, Rabbi Judah raises the theological stakes, rendering the appropriation of Roman capital (thus, legal) practice as a violation of the biblical commandment not to join the idolatrous rites of the Egyptians and the Canaanites. The toseftan Rabbi Judah rejects a Scottian subversive reading of this appropriation, arguing, in Berkowitz's words, that "you cannot be a Rabbi and look like a Roman. . . . Rabbi Judah worries that in the Sages' resistance to Rome they will ultimately come to resemble them. The reversal of power will really be no reversal, since the executioner will look exactly the same."[60] In these passages, the rabbis are contending with the following dilemma: on the one hand, "if rabbinic power is to look nothing like Roman power, then it is not power"; if, on the other hand, "rabbinic power is to look too much like Roman power, then it is not rabbinic."[61]

The rabbis thus face a paradox of power: How, in Berkowitz's words, "do they assert their authority when they have so little of it within the status system of imperial Rome?"[62] In relation to the Roman imperium, they are oppressed, subject, and subaltern, and their discourse around execution grapples with this fact. Yet at the same time, they are attempting to establish themselves as both physical and metaphysical authorities over their fellow Jews, and here, too, their discourse around execution facilitates this. One place this is evident is in the mishnaic account of execution by stoning. Whereas in the Tanakh, priestly accounts of stoning call for the condemned to be pelted with stones by their entire community, and some Deuteronomistic sources call for primary victims or witnesses to initiate the execution (with the community following), the Mishnah, in Sanhedrin 6:4, formalizes the stoning process, giving the primary role as executioner first to one witness, then to a second, and then to the community only if the two witnesses' actions have not proven lethal.[63]

As Berkowitz notes, here "the role of the community as executioner is almost, though not completely, eliminated by the Mishnah."[64] Particularly by elevating the witness as executioner over and above the community as a whole, the rabbis assert far-reaching control over the ritual of execution. Rabbinic law determines who is a legitimate witness, and that law also gives judicial discretion to decide a witness's legitimacy to a rabbinic court.[65] The witness-executioners are further managed by rabbinic restrictions on their actions through the rabbis' very particular interpretations of a specific biblical phrase.[66] The rabbis, as Berkowitz argues, thereby "formalize [execution], hemming in the actions of the witnesses, making them conform to a procedure controlled by *rabbinic exegesis*."[67]

Thus, the defining activity of sagehood—that of the intrarabbinic discursive interpretation of biblical text—becomes, within the tannaitic literary universe, the ultimate authority over rituals of guilt and innocence, life and death, for their imagined community. Particularly as the rabbis grappled with their status as occupied, subaltern, and inescapably influenced by Roman authorities and practices that at least some of them would have preferred to banish, it became crucial that the activity that was most constitutive of their identity wield considerable political, theological, and epistemic power within their own text world. So the ritual of execution, as Berkowitz argues, is "not just about criminals and courts but about the power of the Rabbis to redeem any Jew"—imperial power be damned. So in this complex resistance to imperial authority, the rabbis' complicated social play nevertheless reinforced, reimagined, and reproduced durable hegemonies and hierarchies that had far-reaching implications on multiple levels.

The Matter May Be Compared: Rabbinic Execution Discourse and BDSM as Circuits of Power

The power play of the BDSM dungeon and the execution play of the tannaitic bet midrash both have a complex relationship with the mainstream power structures to which they exist in apparent opposition. The theatrical character of each is key to these complex relations, for both the rabbinic discourse and BDSM practice are forms of theatrical play and imagination. They are, however, far from being "mere" play. Weiss's kinksters' play, despite (and, in part, because of) the rhetoric of its being "just" play, feeds on and contributes to "real-world" dynamics in an ongoing and fluid relationship that Weiss calls a "circuit," which "works when connections are created between realms that are imagined as isolated and opposed."[68] Thus, BDSM space positions itself as doubly separated from the normative sociosexual hierarchies it wants to resist: as queer (that is, sexually transgressive) space such that "all [its] practices are oppositional to heteronormative social institutions" and as play space in which all players may choose, consent to, reverse, or renegotiate their roles and experiences, thus "disrupt[ing] the heterosexual logic that animates sex-gender-sexuality binaries because roles are chosen, rather than naturalized (based on sexed bodies)."[69] In either case, BDSM therefore defines itself as set apart from and in ontological opposition to these normative structures, as a "queer counterpublic."[70] Yet, in delineating these categories of heteronormativity and queerness, of real world and scene, such definitions "can reaffirm a static hierarchy of sex practices based on oppositionality."[71] Thus, in addition to the ways described above in which organized kink can reinforce pernicious hierarchies, Weiss argues, its very rhetoric of dichotomous opposition ensures its continued participation in and dependence on that against which it defines itself. Its own investment in its subversive and transgressive character keeps it in a mutually reinforcing circuit with that which it strives to transgress.

The rabbis' texts, too, are forms of transgressive play that depend on that which they transgress. It is unlikely that the classical rabbis, especially the tannaim, had much real legal authority even within their own communities at the time they were active.[72] It is therefore unlikely that any of the rituals of execution described in these texts were ever carried out as such. Further, each is quite aware of its own theatrical character, although where BDSM practitioners, according to Weiss, overdetermine the theatrical character of their practice to insulate themselves from the full implications of its relationship to oppressive power structures, the rabbis, per Berkowitz, are anxious and ambivalent about the theatrical character of their rituals and seek rhetorical distance from it. This is in large part because the theater and the arena are spaces that are inextricably associated with Greece and Rome.[73] Yet the rituals of execution the rabbis articulate unfold as spectacles that mirror Rome not only in their methods (decapitation by sword) but in their theatricality (precisely choreographed steps, delineated roles, and the community's role as audience). Just as Weiss's kinksters, then, create and sustain circuits between public and private, normativity and transgression, and resistance and reproduction of dominant norms, so too, here, the rabbis create circuits between sage and centurion, Jew and Gentile, Jerusalem and Rome (or Athens), bet midrash and arena.

Thus, although rabbinic discourse and BDSM are forms of imaginative play, they are, despite BDSM's overemphasis on theatrical remove and rabbinic discourse's ambivalence about the same, forms of play that have very real physical, cultural, and political consequences. Even if kinksters position themselves outside of normative social and political discourses, they nevertheless participate in them, generating communities of particular consumers that feed capitalist economies, reenacting the dynamics they seek to upend, and producing, above all, deeply felt emotional and affective responses, direct and indirect, to the scenes they enact. And even if, as is likely, the rabbis never carried out a single one of their richly described rituals of execution, their texts create rabbinic authority going forward by bringing into being a literary and legal world in which the play of text does real work in the world. Indeed, as tannaitic text traveled forward in time to take its central role in Judaism as we know it today, it came to acquire the sort of legal, political, and metaphysical status within halakhic Judaism that it strove for in its composition and redaction. Even though actual acts of execution continued to be beyond the political power of most Jewish communities, the rituals of execution the rabbis described "furnish[ed] a kind of imaginary space for its audience, a space in which rabbinic word and its violent deed were intimately linked."[74] And the sort of power this ritualized text play helped generate meant that the rabbis and their heirs had overwhelming power to define and determine what constituted acceptable Jewish ways of being.

Derive from This: Paths of Potential Correction

Contemplating the discontents of social and communal resistance to regnant power structures such as those I discuss above can leave one who is committed to such subversion feeling as though they are floundering in a tar pit, where every attempt to free oneself leads only to further entrapment. And the comparison I make above seems to offer little help. If neither the rabbis of the second and third centuries nor the kinksters of today can help but reproduce the power structures they seek to transgress, what hope is there?

Weiss claims that BDSM scenes that are truly politically effective "disrupt certain ideological constructs—what I have been calling alibis—that separate the social and the sexual. They suggest that, contrary to community ideology, SM isn't equally available to everyone, an unmarked, universalized practice; rather, racial, gendered, and classed difference is at the center of SM practice."[75] I argue here that one way in which classical rabbinic discourse can correct contemporary BDSM communities is that it is all too aware that it is not open to everyone. The details of this comparison between the tannaim and contemporary kinksters can provide some technologies of mutual correction, ones that may help produce communities and techniques of the social self that are more genuinely inclusive and liberatory. The parallels between the layers of power play that exist within organized BDSM and those evinced by tannaitic execution texts are, I argue, morally productive. Inasmuch as the problematics of rabbinic power serve as a warning to kinksters (and others) who see their play as an escape from the complex power structures they inhabit and reproduce, these texts confirm that such dynamics are far from new. Inasmuch, however, as the rabbis are *aware* of their appropriation of Roman power structures for their own sacred play, this dynamic also serves as a corrective to contemporary players. Conversely, contemporary

players' *rhetorical*, if not always actualized, commitment to diversity and or-
ganizational egalitarianism stands as a corrective to the rabbis' exclusiveness
and authoritarianism. What the rabbis' self-awareness might accomplish,
then, is to aid many contemporary players' attempts to move that commitment further along the path from rhetoric to fact.

Women of color and especially Black women BDSM players model ways
in which a critical awareness of circuits of power can move the moral claims
of BDSM further from theory into conscious political praxis. In her study of
race play (BDSM scenes that eroticize aspects of racialized oppression such
as motifs of US chattel slavery) as performed by Black women in BDSM,
Ariane Cruz argues that these practitioners demonstrate the ways in which,
in their play, "not just racism [is] eroticized, but also a vibrantly imagined
racial difference in which the color line between black and white is *played*
with—constantly smudged, re-delineated, and traversed."[76] Mollenna Williams, one of the most visible and outspoken Black BDSM practitioners and
educators on the contemporary scene and an advocate of race play, states,
"I do race play whether or not I want to."[77] Williams's words, Cruz argues,
"testify to the alreadyness and perdurability of race play for black women . . .
[which] contrasts with the ephemerality of race play for white men, who, as
Weiss notes, know that 'when the scene is done, 'it's done.'"[78] Because, as
Amber Jamilla Musser argues, Williams's race play is so explicitly public,
she "[makes] visible the ways that race and racial histories structure domination and submission and the pleasures they might provide."[79] While, for
Weiss's mostly white informants, the categories of play and fantasy work to
obscure the ways in which BDSM practice is dependent on and productive
of the broader social world, Cruz's subjects are intimately aware of these
relationships and often quite consciously exploit and subvert them; further,
in doing so publicly, they force a broader social confrontation of the painful
and ongoing histories and power structures that prefigure and continue to
undergird their performances.

Disabled and chronically ill practitioners also model this awareness. Here,
one of the most outspoken voices is Bob Flanagan, the "Super Masochist"
who juxtaposes the pain of his cystic fibrosis (CF) and its treatments with
his BDSM play and performance art. Flanagan's performances challenge any
neat separation between scene and "real life": just as Williams "does race play
whether or not [she] wants to," Flanagan did pain whether or not he wanted

to. The pain of masochism is linked to yet distinct from the pain of CF. In *The Pain Journal*, a chronicle of the last year of his life, Flanagan reflects on the ebb and flow of his medical pain and its relationship to his masochism; in an August entry, he is aroused by the sight of fetish gear but too exhausted and ill to follow through.[80] In an April entry, by contrast, he writes, "Last call for Demerol (I wish). Don't need pain killers now. I'm a masochist again!"[81] Masochistic pain is a pain produced by Flanagan's bodily discipline; CF pain is not so controllable. Neither, however, exists in isolation from the other.[82]

Flanagan explicitly disrupts the regnant norm that both the pain of illness and the sensations of sexual play are private, not to be displayed publicly and certainly not to be deliberately displayed so. As Musser writes, "Flanagan challenges the notion of masochism as a private practice by relying on an implicit audience and producing a performance of submission, guilt, or pain."[83] One is not supposed to be sick in public, to be sexual in public, nor to sexualize pain. Sick people are not supposed to be sexual, let alone deviantly so, and they are certainly not supposed to be deviantly sexual in public. Yet Flanagan's work forces the audience to confront ways of being from which they have been insulated and models ways of being and of living with pain that have been foreclosed.[84] He knows that boundaries of public and private, pain and pleasure, sickness and flourishing, are permeable, and he seeks to puncture them further, to lay bare the ways that deviant pains bleed into, shape, and are shaped by the erotic, which in turn bleeds into and shapes the everyday.

The rabbis, too, consciously rupture the boundaries between Roman and Jewish structures, between Roman punishments and Jewish rituals, and between the imaginary Jew condemned by their own courts and the very real Jew martyred by the empire. A passage from the tannaitic midrash Mekhilta D'Rabbi Ishmael reproduces Roman punishments far more explicitly than the mishnaic passages already treated, juxtaposing them with distinctively rabbinic execution methods and linking them all to the martyrdom of righteous Jews:

> R. Natan says: "of those that love Me and keep My commandments" (Ex. 20:5): these are they who dwell in the land of Israel and put forth their lives for the commandments.
>
> Why do you go to be decapitated? Because I circumcised my son to be an Israelite.

Why do you go to be burned? Because I recited from the Torah.
Why do you go to be crucified? Because I ate matzah.
Why are you taking a hundred lashes? Because I shook the lulav.
And it says: "those with which I was wounded in the house of those I love"
(Zech. 13:6)—these caused me to be beloved by my Father in Heaven.[85]

While this passage is in some ways a paradigmatic example of the sort of circuit Weiss describes, in others, as Berkowitz shows, it demonstrates a triumph of the rabbis' performance of interpretive and mimetic reversal. The "distinctively Roman" litany of deaths—it includes crucifixion—also seems to echo the Rabbis' own punishment methods, with its list of four and its executions of decapitation [and] burning. Roman execution, in the Rabbis' representation, comes to resemble the Rabbis own executions."[86] The ordering of Berkowitz's words here is important. In her analysis of mishnaic execution rituals, she treats the rabbis as appropriating Roman ritual such that their own executions come to resemble Rome's. Here, it is reversed: explicitly marked Roman technologies (crucifixion) are forced into a rabbinic formal structure and made to share space with explicitly rabbinic punishments.[87] Further, the Roman punishments in rabbinic structures are made to serve explicitly rabbinic moral, political, and eschatological ends: they enable righteous Jews to give their lives for Torah and so receive ultimate divine reward. Finally, first as recited Oral Torah and then as redacted and disseminated text, the performance of this "reverse mimicry" remains public at a meta level, making apparent both the rabbis' appropriation and their subversion of these explicitly Roman power structures.[88] In this way, Berkowitz argues, "the Rabbis mimic the gradations of Roman executions but at the same time reject the underlying principles of Roman power."[89] We can see parallels to the sort of subversion that occurs in this passage in Flanagan's work, for Flanagan, too, forces the pain of illness and medical treatment into the broader frame of the chosen pain of his masochism, even as he confronts the ways his medical pain inhibits his practice. Williams, likewise, explicitly forces the theatrics of American chattel slavery and racism into a performative frame of her own design.

Berkowitz argues that, by reading these passages through Scott's framework of "hidden transcript," we can see that, rather than being mere play or discourse (not least because these rituals were likely never carried out), the rabbis' clear and ironic awareness (and internal disputation of) their dependence on Roman techniques of power renders their texts understandable "not as a deflection of real action but as the breeding ground for it . . . as *practical* discourse, as real critique."[90] These examples of execution play thus, "in their resistance to Rome and in their disputes about the best way to resist, display the charisma of the Rabbis, in whose conversations the Rabbis hoped the Jews of the Roman Empire would be able to recognize their own concerns."[91] The rabbis display a critical awareness of the circuits of power in which they are enmeshed, and they deploy that awareness to notable effect.

Furthermore, the parallels between the rabbis and contemporary BDSM players demonstrate that the problems inherent in discursive, disciplined risk play within alternative communities and their relationships to hegemonic power structures are neither a solely modern phenomenon nor a phenomenon limited to explicitly sexual activities. If the play of practitioners like Williams and Flanagan productively transgresses boundaries of private and public, play and real life, speakable and unspeakable, the execution play of the rabbis adds a productive transgression of boundaries of then and now, sacred and secular, flesh and text, study and spectacle—and of sexual and nonsexual.

Ultimately, then, the rabbis' best corrective to kinksters comes not from the texts we have treated in this section but from one treated in the previous section: that old chestnut, the tanur shel akhnai. For that text, outlandish as it may seem to modern readers, gives lie to the fantasy articulated by Weiss's kinksters: that text is merely text, that play is merely play, and that either exists in some kind of safe space isolated from the rest of society. Rather, the tanur shel akhnai shows us, to play with text, even concerning the most obscure and mundane detail, is to play with that which organizes and defines the worlds we live in on social, political, environmental, and metaphysical levels. In doing so, it shows us that the risks we heighten and dramatize—whether that occurs in the bet midrash, the dungeon, or the bedroom—are inextricably linked with the risks we navigate throughout our daily lives. To play responsibly with those risks begins with an uncompromising awareness of those connections and continues by bringing that awareness into the ways we form ourselves as moral beings within our communities. If we do that, we perhaps stand a better chance of truly subverting the problematic structures and praxes that invariably feed our own.

By the same token, kinksters' best corrective to the rabbis' legacy, and to our own political and social worlds, comes from their aspirations and ideals. Kinksters imagine a community in which collective affinity and self-discipline is not troubled but rather nourished by diversity—physical, economic, and especially sexual. While their embodied communities may, in practice, often fail to live up to that ideal, in imagining it ,they nevertheless present a script—and, as the rabbis teach us, scripts, as texts, have real normative power—for communities that are both livable and morally constructive for a diversity of members. And both the rabbis and the kinksters, meanwhile, offer the rest of us a corrective in their embrace of risk and their management of the same through negotiation and constant discourse, for—fantasies of separation aside—play is not just play, and talk is not just talk. They are powerful moral techniques that shape us whether we want them to or not.

CONCLUSION

THE ACTIVITIES OF SEX—doing it, talking about it, thinking about it, regulating it—are sites of ongoing moral formation on individual, interpersonal, and communal levels. Putting the various ways those activities form us in careful dialogue with rabbinic texts, all of which pivot around the likewise morally formative activities of communal text study, can help us to identify and nurture the *kinds* of moral formation that contribute to building a world that is kinder, more just, more thoughtful, and more liberating.

In this book, I have identified some of those kinds of moral formation. I have, throughout, discussed ways that sex, especially in dialogue with classical rabbinic texts, helps us think about the virtues of empirical justice, hermeneutic competency, wise risk management, and diverse interdependence. All these virtues are applicable in nonsexual social situations as well. Hermeneutic competency as a moral norm has critical implications for medicine, politics, and education. Wise risk management and its component virtues already draw a great deal on lessons from disability studies and activism, and thinking about risk in these ways can, in turn, help break down systemic ableism, as well as other bigotries that cast minoritized groups as less entitled to the dignity of risk while simultaneously painting them as embodying risks themselves. Diverse interdependence might bespeak a way forward for groups and communities that seek to navigate a broader culture that encourages assimilation, allowing them to adapt to and accommodate the ways their members are changing while maintaining a sense of collective identity and holding on to those ways in which that collective identity shapes members toward livable, constructive, and, where applicable, holy ends.

I conclude this book with one more rabbinic story, one that, in one way or another, demonstrates the importance of these virtues. Unlike the other texts I have treated, this story, from Kidushin 81b, actually does have sex as its subject matter, and so I engage it with caution, because to a great extent I think that what I have claimed generally about explicitly sexual rabbinic texts—that they are not, ultimately or most interestingly, about sex—holds true here as well. Here, as elsewhere, rabbinic sex isn't about sex so much as it is about self-mastery, about sex as a site for the cultivation of exemplary sagely control. The immediate context of the story—it is prefaced by a series of tempted sage narratives and followed by a discussion of the role of intent in moral action—underscores this reading. As with the story of Rav Kahana under his master's bed that I discussed in chapter 1, the story I treat here should not be read as evidence that the Talmud is somehow sex positive.

At the same time, some judicious counterreading can highlight aspects of this text that draw out some key themes I have addressed throughout this book. Primary among these is the sense that the protagonists' sexual behaviors and self-formations, for good and for ill, are not unrelated to their nonsexual social characters. The way the characters form themselves sexually seems to have a lot to do with the way they form themselves in other ways, most notably in how they communicate with one another and interpret—or ignore!—the other's communication. We can read this story as showing us that interpretive skill—hermeneutic competency!— is just as important in sexual and more broadly social interactions as it is in an immediately rabbinic context. But it also shows us that interpretive skill in one area is not enough to help us in others if we are not attentive to these interconnections.

We encounter the story of Rabbi Ḥiyya bar Ashi and his wife after a series of tempted sage narratives. In all but the first of the preceding cases, the sage is incautious in his speech, either mocking those who give in to the evil inclination or, in the final case, mocking the personified evil inclination itself. In each case, the sage is then chastened when he is exposed to a temptation he cannot resist—a sexual temptation in the first two cases and a temptation to shame and ridicule in the final one. So we enter the story primed to think, in some way, about hubris and the dangers of undiscerning speech.

R. Ḥiyya's story seems to start out in a more promising fashion. He doesn't seem to assume that he is too righteous to give in to the *yetser hara*, instead regularly praying for deliverance from it. But then, something interesting happens when the text reveals that the point-of-view character is not R. Ḥiyya but his wife:

> It was Rabbi Ḥiyya bar Ashi's habit, every time he would fall on his face, to say, "May the merciful one deliver us from the yetser hara!"
> One day, his wife heard him.[1] She said, "Now, it's been goodness knows *how* many years since he's separated himself from me. So what is the reason he says this?"

We learn from R. Ḥiyya's wife that she and her husband have not had sex in years, something that, as her subsequent actions will indicate, seems to make her less than pleased. But overhearing his prayer reveals to her that his failure to have sex with her—something, by the way, that he is halakhically obligated to do!—is not due to a diminished libido or to impotence.[2] R. Ḥiyya's *yetser ra* has not left him. He simply does not direct it toward her.

Notice that from the very beginning of the story, matters are framed in terms of habitual action and the formation of the self. R. Ḥiyya's specific prayer is explicitly described as a habit, and it, in turn, is part of a broader habit of daily supplication. From his wife, we then learn of another habit of his: he no longer has sex with her. And we can infer yet another habit from this exchange: given that his wife has to piece these things together from overhearing his prayer, R. Ḥiyya does not seem to be in the habit of discussing his decisions with his wife—which in and of itself indicates his failure to practice the virtues I've discussed throughout this book. He is not practicing diverse interdependence or, indeed, human interdependence of any kind. Nor is he practicing empirical justice: *doing the damn research* includes listening to the people who have a stake in the question at hand. He isn't practicing wise risk management: clearly, he sees his yetser hara as dangerous, but instead of working out how to mitigate the most problematic elements of it, he's praying for it to just go away. Finally, all of this indicates he isn't demonstrating hermeneutic competency—he seems to have fundamentally misread the way his yetser hara works, the ways this affects his wife, and, in turn, what that implies about how he should respond to it.

R. Ḥiyya has, through daily practice, shaped his bodily and mental conduct in particular directions. He does so, presumably, under the impression that these ways of being are good and righteous. But are they? R. Ḥiyya's wife is, we can imagine, both frustrated and curious, and she decides to figure out what is going on—she decides, in other words, to do the damn research. She disguises herself and seeks him out while he is at yet another habit, that of study:

> One day, while he was studying in his garden, she adorned herself and repeatedly sashayed before him.
> He said to her: who are you?
> She said to him: I am Ḥaruta, and I'm just returning today.
> He propositioned her.
> She said to him: Bring me that pomegranate from the top branch. He sprung up, went, and brought it to her.

R. Ḥiyya's wife successfully disguises herself from her husband, offering him the moniker "Ḥaruta." She successfully entices him to have sex with her as she could not when presenting as his wife.

There's quite a bit going on in this section of the story, but there are two aspects to which I want to give particular attention. First, what R. Ḥiyya is doing when his wife approaches him is worth unpacking. I've already noted that we can read it through the frame of the story's opening as one more habit of R. Ḥiyya's. But what kind of habit is it? The word translated here as "studying," *gereis*, has the more basic sense of "collecting" or "accumulating." R. Ḥiyya is studying by himself, here, rather than engaging in the social activity of interpreting and debating in the bet midrash, and he is, as Marcus Jastrow renders the root here, "committing traditions to memory," learning by rote rather than interpreting.[3] We've already seen that R. Ḥiyya doesn't seem to be in the habit of discussing important information with his wife; it is notable here that when she encounters him doing the activity that most fully constitutes his identity and character as a rabbi, he is also doing it alone, without discussion. Granted, the bet midrash was an all-male space—narratively speaking, she can't approach him in there. But the parallel between his conduct here and his conduct with his wife is nevertheless striking, and it points to his failure to do empirical justice to his wife—both regarding his sexual relationship with her and to her own broader agency and self-accounting.

Second, R. Ḥiyya's wife's actions here are also important. To begin with, it is here that she does for herself what the text will not do for her: she names herself. A woman who takes initiative in naming herself can also take sexual initiative, and she does so. Here, too, sex and communication are intimately linked. This is true of nonverbal communication as it is of verbal; not only the name she gives herself but the visual cues she adopts—dressing herself in a way that says "pay attention to me!" and repeatedly walking in front of her husband—also form a character that grasps and exercises her sexual, social, and moral agency. And we should also note the parallel between R. Ḥiyya's various forms of repeated, habitual action and Ḥaruta's repeated action of passing before him. R. Ḥiyya's habits have primed him not to engage with her; she therefore takes a repeated action to break his habit of disengagement.

The name she offers, Ḥaruta, is also significant: as Gail Labovitz notes, it could share a root, her, with the word ḥerut, or "freedom."[4] This is notable in light of a regnant reading of the character of Ḥaruta as a prostitute: in the ancient world, sex work would have been one of a woman's few paths to economic freedom. However, the name could also refer to a root, ḥeret, with valences meaning "dried up, shrunk," or "engraven."[5] This name might be read as risk contained in a single word: Ḥaruta has announced herself a free agent. Will R. Ḥiyya relate to her honestly and directly, moral agent to moral agent? Or will he fail to engage and shrivel up? Either way, what happens will be engraved, recorded, remembered.

> When he came home, his wife was kindling the oven. He went up and sat inside it.[6]
> She said to him: What is this?
> He said to her: Thus and such an incident happened.
> She said to him: It was I.
> He paid her no mind until she brought him signs.
> He said to her: Regardless, I intended something forbidden.

The answer comes soon enough. When R. Ḥiyya returns from the garden, Ḥaruta has resumed her domestic role, and R. Ḥiyya continues not to engage, even treating the oven that she has painstakingly kindled—working with wood-fired ovens is hard labor!—as an instrument for his own increasingly extreme askesis. Ḥaruta, however, continues to embrace communicative agency and questions him. He then relates what he believes has occurred, and at this point Ḥaruta reveals the ruse to her husband, explaining that his actions were entirely licit.

But R. Ḥiyya is too absorbed in his own ruminations to pay attention to her words or to her herself as a speaker—again failing to do the situation empirical justice and failing to demonstrate even rudimentary hermeneutic competency. She must bring visual signs before he even acknowledges her basic descriptive account—but even then, he fails to acknowledge, let alone try to understand, her moral accounting. Instead of engaging the moral agent who stands before him, he is overcome with guilt at what he sees as his own failure to overcome temptation—a temptation, evidently, that he feared enough to desist even from the sexual activities in which he was not only allowed but actually commanded to engage. And in so doing, he also fails to engage his wife as a sexual, social, and moral actor in her own right.

The story's coda confirms, at last, that R. Ḥiyya has indeed chosen shriveling over freedom. He responds to Ḥaruta's revelation with even greater physical self-abnegation, eventually fasting to the point that he dies of starvation: "All of the days of that righteous man, he would fast, until he died by that very death." So much for wise risk management: R. Ḥiyya has taken an all-or-nothing approach to the risk of his yetser hara; since he hasn't been delivered from it, he might as well die. Thus passes the glory of extreme askesis. And while the Gemara itself seems subsequently to support R. Ḥiyya's moral accounting that his intent mattered above all else, in this counterreading, one might, instead, carefully draw the lesson that poor communication—sexual, social, interpretive—kills.

The context of this story wants us to think about it in terms of sagely self-control and askesis. Even a counterreading that privileges Ḥaruta's perspective, I believe, makes it about sex only inasmuch as sex is a site for thinking about the moral import of clear and honest communication with those with whom one has any kind of socially intimate relationship. It is thus in the ways that this text is *not* primarily about sex that it is instructive for our own sexual ethics. And yet at the same time, it demonstrates how thinking well about sex is one important part of thinking about social interaction more generally and how failure to think well about sex can indicate poor social thinking elsewhere—how, in the end, sex is not so neatly separable from the rest of our lives.

So what do we learn from all this? Throughout, I have argued that if we are to take seriously the claim that sex is a species of social intercourse, we need to understand the extent of that claim's implications for normative sexual ethics. And one significant implication is this: if sex is a species of social intercourse, it follows from this that the study of sex can teach us a great deal about social ethics more generally. This means that all ethicists, whether or not we specifically focus on sex and sexuality, would do well to pay particular and serious attention to sex as a moral category. We are leaky, ridiculous, vulnerable, mortal, pleasure-seeking beings navigating a world in which risk is at once ubiquitous and important to livability, pleasure is polymorphous, many kinds of intimate interaction—some unexpected—are commonplace, and our distinct, unique, idiosyncratic selves are inextricably bound up in complex webs of collective dependencies and duties with one another. Sex as a social phenomenon touches all of these issues, and thinking with and about sex—and doing it well—is incredibly helpful for understanding some of what they mean for how we should strive to act in such a world.

Throughout this book I have claimed, perhaps paradoxically, that sex should not, either descriptively or prescriptively speaking, be cordoned off from other forms of social interaction and that sex in particular has something to teach us about social ethics more broadly. How can I claim both? Perhaps it is best to say that it is precisely because we have so often tended to cordon sex off from the rest of our sociality that its teachings for us have gone unexplored. In making sex, as Eve Kosofsky Sedgwick has put it, "in modern Western culture the most meaning-intensive of human activities," modern Western ethics has, ironically, lost access to some of the really interesting possible meanings of the fact that most adult humans will at some point in their lives seek pleasure and express social and emotional connection through some form of mutual contact and exposure.[7] If we can do the damn research—if we can do sex proper empirical justice and think about what happens during these mutual exposures, especially among those individuals and communities that regnant power structures have shunned for their sexualities—we might find some important moral instruction on how to do all kinds of mutual exposures in ways that are more thoughtful, humane, and even reparative.

Can sex in and of itself solve entrenched harms, oppressions, and power disparities? Of course not. Sex, like any other interaction, is only one part of how we form and express ourselves as moral agents. I thus agree with Patrick Califia when he says that sex does not "have an inherent power to transform the world"—indeed, no one thing does!—and that we cannot "fuck our way to freedom."[8] I do, however, believe that by forcing ourselves to understand sexuality and its inextricable relationship to the rest of our social world better, we can begin through that understanding to transform the world. Sex is intricately bound up with and productive of power, identity, and health, and it will prove difficult to repair these relationships if we are not capable of speaking frankly about, let alone beginning to understand, the roles our bodily desires play in producing them. By studying in greater detail the moral relationships between our sexual lives and the other parts of our social lives, we can help create the world of open discourse about sex and risk that is modeled by the mishnaic conversation on ritual impurity and by the risk-conditioned community of the literary bet midrash, and we can also come to a better understanding of ourselves as social and moral beings.

NOTES

Introduction

1. Rachel Adler, for example, in *Engendering Judaism: An Inclusive Theology and Ethics*, focuses largely on rereading texts to come up with a portrait of a holy and egalitarian sexuality that lays a groundwork for thinking about sexually charged relationships in general but does not answer questions about how to navigate particular sexual situations or manage problems that might arise in even the most egalitarian of contexts. Similarly, Judith Plaskow (with coauthor Donna Berman), even in *The Coming of Lilith: Essays on Feminism, Judaism, and Sexual Ethics, 1972–2003*, a book that is in part about sexual ethics, ends up offering very little in the way of specific normative guidance. This gap becomes even starker when we add engagement with *halakhah* to the equation. Relatively progressive figures in post-halakhic traditions, like the Reform and Reconstructionist movements, have shown a willingness to be practical and broadly normative (if not necessarily systematic) about their sexual ethics, but since they do not see themselves as bound in any significant way by the halakhic tradition, their path toward affirming unconventional sexual behavior is much easier. More recently, Jewish feminists like Danya Ruttenberg, editor of and contributor to *The Passionate Torah: Sex and Judaism*, have begun to give some serious attention to Jewish sexual ethics from a perspective that is both halakhically engaged and interested in navigating specific practical problems. As yet, however, this promising work has appeared as collections of shorter essays rather than as any kind of systemic, book-length treatment.

One exception to this trend is Jennie Rosenfeld's dissertation, "Talmudic Rereadings: Toward a Modern Orthodox Sexual Ethic." Rosenfeld reads Talmudic and Hasidic texts through a lens of critical theory to move toward an ethic of sanctifying sexual experiences while "owning one's actions" (330). Together with

David S. Ribner, Rosenfeld is also the author of *Et Le'ehov: The Newlywed's Guide to Sexual Intimacy*, a sex manual aimed at modern Orthodox married couples that is groundbreaking in its candor and relatively expansive attitude toward sexual pleasure.

2. See, for just a few examples, Borowitz, *Choosing a Sex Ethic*, 107; Lamm, *Jewish Way in Love*; Bulka, *Jewish Marriage*; Dorff, *Love Your Neighbor* and "Jewish Perspective on Birth Control"; and Novak, *Jewish Social Ethics*, among cautious or restrictive voices; and Ruttenberg, *Passionate Torah*; Teutsch, *Guide to Jewish Practice*; and Green, "Contemporary Approach," among expansive or permissive voices.

3. See Raucher, "Ethnography and Jewish Ethics," for a pointed critique of this overreliance and for a proposed model for ethnographic sources as an alternative foundation for doing Jewish ethics.

4. Hamraie, *Building Access*, 12.

5. Hamraie, 12.

6. I say "pregnancy" rather than specifying "unwanted pregnancy" here because even wanted pregnancies are physically and psychologically risky undertakings in their own right. In fact, this in and of itself is one example of my broader point: the "right" pregnancies (wanted pregnancies undertaken by married women between the ages of about twenty and thirty-five) are still demonstrably risky undertakings, and yet we consider them worthwhile enough that we do not see assuming their risks as foolhardy or irresponsible.

7. Steven Greenberg, *Wrestling With God and Men: Homosexuality in the Jewish Tradition*, 12.

8. Though, as Margot Weiss, in *Techniques of Pleasure: BDSM and the Circuits of Sexuality* convincingly argues, the BDSM practitioners who were her informants, and even many of the classic scholars in the fields of queer, feminist, and sexuality studies (notably, Michel Foucault) maintain a certain fantasy that sex, especially queer or otherwise transgressive sex, is somehow separated from the "real world." (loc. 6, 17) See, for example, Foucault, "Sexual Choice, Sexual Act," 322–34; Karmen MacKendrick, *Counterpleasures*; Jeremy R. Carrette, "Intense Exchange: Sadomasochism, Theology, and the Politics of Late Capitalism," 11–30.

9. Nussbaum, "'Whether from Reason.'"

10. Analogy to professional athletes suggested by Margaret Mohrmann in a seminar in the spring of 2012 while discussing Nussbaum's argument. Analogy to clergy suggested by Rabbi Ruti Regan, personal correspondence, August 7, 2018.

11. The International Labour Organization's 2017 global report estimates that, globally, 16 million people are forced to labor in private industries, of which 24 percent were in domestic labor, 18 percent in construction, 15 percent in manufacturing, and 11 percent in fishing and agriculture. The same report estimates that 3.8 million adults and 1 million children are in forced sexual labor. It's also worth noting that all of these statistics are blurry at best, owing both to the clandestine

nature of forced labor and to organizations' dependence on numbers provided by NGOs whose definitions and models of what constitutes "trafficking" influence the quantitative data they collect in a range of ways. See for example Goodey, "Human Trafficking," and Chuang, "Rescuing Trafficking."

12. Gaca, *Making of Fornication*, 92.

13. Gaca, 94.

14. Gaca, 176; see, for example, the extended metaphor in Hosea.

15. Gaca, 180.

16. On this, see also the classic studies Brown, *Body and Society*; and Rouselle, *Porneia*.

17. See Lacquer, *Making Sex*.

18. Gaca, chap. 3. And, again, note the similarity to contemporary anti-sex-work prejudice.

19. MacIntyre, *After Virtue*, 64.

20. McRuer, *Crip Theory*; Sandahl, "Queering the Crip"; Kafer, *Feminist, Queer, Crip*.

21. Balberg, *Purity, Body, and Self*.

22. Rubenstein, *Culture of the Babylonian*; Schofer, *Making of a Sage*.

23. Berkowitz, *Execution and Invention*, 154, 162–65; J. Scott, *Domination and the Arts*, 4.

24. Cruz, *Color of Kink*; Musser, *Sensational Flesh*.

25. Rubin, "Thinking Sex."

1. Textual Intercourse

1. Significant parts of this chapter also appear in my 2018 article "Textual Relationships: On Perspective, Interpretive Discipline, and Constructive Ethics." Some parts were also delivered in slightly modified form as a lecture at Washington University in St. Louis on September 14, 2017.

2. For more detail, see my article, "Is Judaism 'Sex Positive'? Understanding Trends in Recent Jewish Sexual Ethics." See also Sarah Imhoff's excellent essay "Jews, Sex Positivity, and Abuse" for a discussion of the potentially harmful consequences of an uncritical rhetoric of Jewish sex positivity.

3. Filler, "Classical Rabbinic Literature," 1. But cf. Raucher, "Ethnography and Jewish Ethics," for a feminist critique of this near ubiquity.

4. Newman, "Woodchoppers and Respirators," 141.

5. Newman, 141.

6. Berkowitz, *Execution and Invention*, 49.

7. Berkowitz, 30, referring to Samuel Mendelsohn's *The Criminal Jurisprudence of the Jews*. Berkowitz notes that these characterizations of the rabbinic stance as either abolitionist or pro death penalty (and as, in either case, notably enlightened

in its stance on the matter) have significant rhetorical force in both intra-Jewish disputes and in discourse between Jews and non-Jews. Mendelsohn, for example, is addressing both Jewish critics of the Talmud who saw rabbinism as an irrational distraction from the "pure" ideals of the Hebrew Bible and "Christian supercessionist criticisms of rabbinic Judaism that it represent[ed] a desiccated form of religion in comparison with its biblical heritage and that heritage's apparent Christian successor" (28). The parallel to the set of rhetorical claims common among contemporary Jewish writers that the rabbinic tradition is deeply and thoroughly sex positive, as opposed to "sex-negative" Christianity or "depraved" secular values, should be clear. It would seem that the practice of making sweeping claims about the stance of "the rabbis" on contemporary ethical problems may be as much a rhetorical response to the challenges of modernity as it is a hermeneutical commitment for its own sake.

    8. Berkowitz, 61.

    9. Berkowitz, 63.

    10. Berkowitz, 70.

    11. The division between Jewish and "other" Western attitudes about men's and women's respective sex drives is hardly so clear-cut. See Satlow, Brown, Rouselle, and others.

    12. Dorff, *Love Your Neighbor*, chap. 3.

    13. Dorff, chap. 3.

    14. I am reminded of a time when, as a rather mediocre student of German, I attempted to render the English expression "I'm cheap"—that is, "I'm stingy" or "penurious"—with the German phrase *Ich bin billig.* After my host mother stopped laughing, she informed me that while the word *billig* might literally mean "inexpensive," I had in fact said something more like "I'm a cheap lay."

    15. Based on a source-critical reading, Michael Satlow in *Tasting the Dish: Rabbinic Rhetorics of Sexuality* traces the overall ambivalence toward sexuality of the rabbinic corpus to a difference between Palestinian and Babylonian sources (especially chap. 6, 7, and 8). By contrast, in *Carnal Israel: Reading Sex in Talmudic Culture,* Daniel Boyarin treats rabbinic anthropology as deeply and fundamentally corporeal; to the extent that he recognizes ascetic threads in rabbinic literature, he ascribes them to Hellenic influence—which, along with Satlow, he sees as more pronounced within Palestinian source material. But, unlike Satlow, he limits this tendency to tannaitic Palestinian sources, whereas Satlow maintains that significant differences along these lines endure between Palestinian and Babylonian Amoraic material, as well. Boyarin, *Carnal Israel,* 35, 47.

    16. Michael Satlow argues that the recognition of sexual pleasure, particularly female sexual pleasure, as a good of sex is nearly unique to Babylonian source material; Palestinian source material, conversely, tends to discuss the goods of sex almost exclusively in terms of procreation. See Satlow, *Tasting the Dish,* 290–94.

17. *Onah* also carries the more specific meaning of "cohabitation," but the texts in question, perhaps in an instance of creating a problem in order to solve it, "interpret onah, literally as 'time'" and from there take it to refer to time-specific sexual obligations. See Satlow, 265–68. Also see b. Yevamot 62b: "R. Yehoshua b. Levi said, any man who knows that his wife fears heaven, and he does not visit her [euphemistic here for sexual relations] is called a sinner, as it is said, 'you shall know that all is well in your tent, when you visit your dwelling [understood here as including your wife,] you shall not sin' (Job 5:24)."

18. Also see Mekhilta Mishpatim 3.

19. Y. Ketubot 5:8 and B. Ketubot 61b–62b, respectively. See Satlow, *Tasting the Dish*, 269–78, for a discussion of these sugyot.

20. See Y. Ketubot 5:10 and B. Ketubot 64b.

21. Satlow, *Tasting the Dish*, 158.

22. See T. Kiddushin 5:9–10 and 5:14, Y. Sotah 1:3, B. Kiddushin 80b–81b.

23. Boyarin, *Carnal Israel*, 47.

24. Lit., "Mother Peace."

25. The appeal to the eugenic value of sexual asceticism is found in several places in rabbinic literature. It was commonly accepted in the ancient world that the circumstances of a child's conception would influence their physical formation, and the rabbinic world was no exception. Directly prior to the dialogue cited above, R. Yohanan b. Dahavei argues that congenital birth defects come as a result of improper marital behavior. B. Pesachim 112b includes a statement that having sex by candlelight will result in epileptic children. Indeed, both the Bavli (Niddah 16b–17a) and the Yerushalmi (Niddah 2:3) forbid sex during the day or by candlelight on grounds of modesty as well as those of eugenics. For more on this, see Satlow, *Tasting the Dish*, 302–14, and especially Neis, *Sense of Sight*.

26. See B. Shabbat 30a, Y. Ketubot 5:8, B. Moed Katan 8b, Y. Moed Katan 1:7.

27. B. Niddah 13a–b. Satlow's excursus on this sugya's redactional structure and the exact point at which the concern over wasted seed was linked to the Mishnah's prohibition on self-arousal is worth perusing. Satlow, *Tasting the Dish*, 246–62.

28. See, for example, Ruttenberg, "Jewish Sexual Ethics."

29. I am indebted to my colleagues and students in the JTS Fellowship in Educating for Applied Jewish Wisdom for many of these insights concerning the Rav Kahana passage and its context; in particular, a havruta session with Rachel Brodie and Lizzi Heydemann was very illuminating.

30. See, variously, Boyarin, *Carnal Israel* and *Unheroic Conduct*; Schofer, *Making of a Sage* and *Confronting Vulnerability*; Alexander, *Gender and Timebound Commandments*.

31. Normatively behaving women, anyway. When women are sexual tempters who serve to test sagely control, they seem to develop rather notable voices indeed.

32. See, for example, Stone, "In Pursuit"; Dorff, "Judaism"; Broyde, "Foundations of Law"; S. Levine, "Capital Punishment"; Colan, "Supreme Court's Talmudic Debate"; Hayes and Israel-Vleeschhouwer, *Jewish Law*. See also Novak, *Jewish Justice*, for examples of broader political-ethical arguments about the influence and continuing applicability of classical Jewish text and reasoning to present-day Western political thought, although to my mind many of these broader claims fall prey to the same sorts of pitfalls I treat here.

33. See, for example, Julia Watts Belser's "Brides and Blemishes: Queering Women's Disability in Rabbinic Marriage Law" for a particularly well-done example of this. Such deliberate counterreading is also a stock in trade of a certain period in Daniel Boyarin's work, although he flags this practice less carefully and explicitly than does Belser.

34. Filler, "Classical Rabbinic Literature," 4.

35. Filler, 5.

36. Filler, 5.

37. Filler, 2. For some examples of how this methodology might be put into practice, see Pava, *Jewish Ethics* and several of the essays in Cutter, *Midrash and Medicine*.

38. Berkowitz, *Execution and Invention*, 63.

39. My use of the terms "functionalist" and "functionalism" ought not be confused with the school of thought in philosophy of mind that specifically defines *mental states* according to their function rather than their structure. Similarly, Filler's account of formalism ought not be confused with the theory of legal formalism, according to which legal rules should be applied to cases without regard for social or political concerns.

40. This is a pitfall to which the formalist approach can still be vulnerable. For example, one formal feature of rabbinic texts that may be quite appealing for ethicists, and which I myself have invoked (see Levi, "Polyvocal Body"), is the polyvocal character of rabbinic discourse. However, the actual extent of this polyvocality is a matter that is very much in dispute among rabbinic scholars, especially regarding halakhic midrash (see, e.g., Dohrman, "Reading as Rhetoric"; and Yadin, *Scripture as Logos*) but even the Talmud (see Boyarin, *Socrates*).

41. I am grateful to Elizabeth Shanks Alexander for suggesting the "source" and "target" framework.

42. Berkowitz, *Execution and Invention*, 20.

43. Kepnes, *Text as Thou*, 58.

44. Kepnes, 69. Kepnes here is referencing Hans Georg Gadamer's concept of the "fusion of horizons," according to which the process of understanding requires coming to an agreement about the context and character of the matter at issue, as well as a common framework or language for engaging it, thereby integrating and taming the strangeness and tension of the encounter. See Gadamer, *Truth and Method*, 301–6.

45. Kepnes, 69.

46. Kepnes, 75.

47. Kepnes, 57.

48. Balberg, *Purity, Body, and Self,* 123.

49. Balberg, 124.

50. Balberg, 138.

51. See Hayes, *Gentile Impurities.* Hayes argues that the analogy between Gentiles and zavim across the tannaitic corpus is partial or incomplete: "Sifra perek Zavim 1:1 and T. Zav 2:1 both indicate that *qodashim* (holy things) are not burned after contact with a Gentile, as they would be after contact with a genuine *zav.* We may assume, therefore, that Gentiles are not"—contrary to the explicit statement in the Tosefta—"deemed to defile like biblical *zavim* in every respect" (124). Hayes further notes that tannaitic sources treat the general presumption of Gentile impurity inconsistently: some sources depict Gentiles interacting with Jews in ways that are explicit routes of impurity transmission, yet no mention is made of any actual impurity, while others specifically mention impurity or defilement occurring as a consequence of such interaction. Hayes speculates that the tannaim distinguished between "sympathetic and hostile Gentiles" (143) and that the major function of the rabbis' system of Gentile impurity "appears to have been the delineation of (perhaps, a reminder of the need for) a barrier between Jews and Gentiles whose intentions were hostile or threatening in some way" (143). This reading, however, seems to cast a moral inflection on the state of impurity itself: "hostile" Gentiles transmit impurity, while "sympathetic" Gentiles do not. Such a direct link between contagion and moral intent seems incongruent with the tannaitic placement of the moral locus of impurity discourse in the careful navigation and management of the impurity-laden world.

52. Balberg, *Purity, Body, and Self,* 140.

53. Balberg, 141.

54. Balberg, 141.

55. Balberg, 145.

56. Balberg, 153.

57. Balberg, 153.

58. Translation in Balberg, 154.

59. M. Ṭaharot 3:8.

60. Balberg, *Purity, Body, and Self,* 155.

61. Balberg, 172. See, for example, M. Ṭaharot 7:4—discussed above regarding the inattentiveness of the amei ha'arets—where "the Rabbis contrasted a woman who is lax in regard to purity with a woman who is stringent in regard to purity by identifying the former as 'the wife of [one of] the People of the Land' (*eshet am ha'arets*) and the latter as 'the wife of a member' (*eshet ḥaver*)."

62. Balberg, 171–72.

63. Balberg, 173.

64. This distinction comes from the same prepositional discrepancy between Lev. 15:2, "When any man has a discharge *mivśaro*," and Lev. 15:19, "When a woman has a discharge of blood *bivśarah*." See Fonrobert, *Menstrual Purity*, 43–56, for a fuller explanation of how the rabbis developed this prepositional discrepancy into an extensive architectural metaphor for female sexual difference.

65. Fonrobert, 103.

66. Mishnah Niddah 2:6–7:

> Five kinds of blood from a woman are impure: the red, the black, like saffron, like water over earth, and like mixed wine.
>
> Bet Shammai say: also like fenugreek water, and like the juice from roasted meat. But Bet Hillel say these are pure.
>
> The green—Akavya ben Mahalalel declared it impure, but the sages declared it pure.
>
> Rabbi Meir said, even if it does not convey impurity by way of a stain, it conveys impurity because it is a liquid. Rabbi Yose said, it is not so in either case.
>
> What is meant by "red"? Like the blood from a wound.
>
> "Black" is like ink; if it is darker than this, it is impure, and if lighter than this, it is pure.
>
> "Like saffron"—the brightest of it.
>
> "Like water over earth"—from the valley of Bet Kerem, and water floats [on top of it].
>
> "Like mixed wine"—two parts water, and one of wine, from the wine of Sharon.

67. Fonrobert, *Menstrual Purity*, 111.

68. Fonrobert, 115.

69. Alexander, "Ancient Jewish Gender," 189.

70. Halberstam, *Law and Truth*, 35.

71. Halberstam, 34.

72. Fonrobert, 112–15. See also her discussion of B. Niddah 57a (pp. 70–82), in which an argument that appears to give some interpretive force to the bleeding woman's physical sensations is systematically neutralized.

73. Halberstam, *Law and Truth*, 39.

74. See Balberg, *Purity, Body, and Self*, 153.

2. Social Intercourse

1. For various articulations of and excurses on the basic claim that sex is a social relation, see, among many others Rubin, "Thinking Sex"; Butler, *Bodies that Matter*; Muñoz, *Cruising Utopia*; Reid-Pharr, *Black Gay Man*; D'Emilio, *Sexual Politics, Sexual Communities*; Martin, "Sexual Practice"; and Elliston, "Anthropology's Queer Future."

2. Rubin, 277.

3. Lorde, "Uses of the Erotic," 53–59, loc. 54.

4. Weiss, *Techniques of Pleasure*, 6.

5. Weiss, 6. See Nelson, *Embodiment*.

6. "Sensual pleasure" replaces "voluptuosity," which is the word for the French *volupté* that appears in Alphonso Lingis's translation. Substitution suggested by Martin Kavka.

7. Levinas, *Totality and Infinity*, 264–65.

8. Berkovits, "Jewish Sexual Ethics," 103–28, loc. 124.

9. Jennie Rosenfeld's dissertation, which is unfortunately unpublished, is a notable exception to this claim. This work is important, especially as it is attentive to Orthodox Jews' needs and moral and ritual commitments in a way that this volume is not and cannot be.

10. Berkovits, "Jewish Sexual Ethics," 124.

11. Berkovits, 124.

12. Berkovits, 114.

13. Plato, for example, classes the desires for food, drink, and sex together under the rubric of appetite (*Republic*, 436a11–b1, 439d8). The Bavli, in Nedarim 20b, compares the rules governing a man's sexual conduct with his wife to those governing consumption of food; note Aline Rouselle at several points discusses the deep connections between dietary and sexual askesis in the classical world and in early Christianity. Rouselle, *Porneia*. In modern philosophy, Bertrand Russell in *Marriage and Morals* argues that sex, like food and drink, is "a natural need" and that "we do not blame a man for a normal and healthy enjoyment of a reasonable quantity of food" (289). Thomas Nagel and Robert Gray both use food as a lens through which to think about the concept of sexual perversion. Nagel, "Sexual Perversion" (1969), and Gray, "Sex and Sexual Perversion" (1978), are both reprinted in Halwani and Soble, *Philosophy of Sex*, 39–52 and 73–84, respectively. There are, likewise, countless examples of visual art, literature, music, and film juxtaposing food and sex and even using food to stand in for more explicit sexuality—consider the famous food fight scene in *Fried Green Tomatoes* (1991) between Idgie and Ruth, a scene that, according to the director Jon Avnet in the DVD commentary, was meant to stand in for sex between the two characters.

14. Fletcher, *Charlemagne's Tablecloth*, 77.

15. Brown Douglas, *Sexuality and the Black Church*, 129.

16. Lorde, "Uses of the Erotic," 56.

17. Brown Douglas, "Black and Blues," 127–28.

18. Sandel, *Liberalism and the Limits*, 173.

19. Sandel, 150.

20. Zoloth, *Healthcare and the Ethics*, 122.

21. Chow, "Politics of Admittance," 57–58.

22. Chow, 58.

23. Chow, 62.

24. Chow, 69.

25. Chow, 74, quoting Bal, *Lethal Love*, 36.

26. Chow, 64.

27. Rubin, "Thinking Sex," 283.

28. Rubin, 280–81.

29. *Lost Girl*, season 3, episode 4, "Fae-de to Black," at 0:43, for the academically curious reader.

In many ways, *Lost Girl*, campy and pulpy as it was, was groundbreaking in its treatment of sex and sexuality. The show revolves around Bo, a bisexual succubus who feeds off her partners' sexual energy. Bo must learn to overcome her sexual guilt, manage the dangerous aspects of her sexual power, and grapple with the ethics of using sex to navigate and lubricate fraught social and political environments. The show treated casual sex, monogamy, and sexual fluidity with surprising nuance. For example, in the above-mentioned episode, Bo must come to terms with the fact that, despite her love for her partner, Lauren, she physically cannot sustain herself off of only one person's sexual energy, driving home the message that not everyone should be—or, indeed, *can be*—monogamous.

30. Rich, "Compulsory Heterosexuality."

31. Ghomeshi was acquitted of sexual assault charges by a Toronto court; his accusers, however, maintain their claims. It is, as always, important to note that legal acquittal in sexual assault cases is far from proof positive that the accused assaulter did not commit the assault. See Stoeffel, "Jian Ghomeshi." See also Spencer, "What I Know About"; Sarah Seltzer, "Feminist BDSM Expert"; Marcotte, "Jian Ghomeshi Accusations"; and Corvid, "Dear Jian Ghomeshi," among other commentaries.

32. MacIntyre, *After Virtue*, 64.

33. MacIntyre, 64.

34. MacIntyre, 63.

35. Leaving aside, for our current purposes, the ages-old debate about whether there is such a thing as a "unity of the virtues" (although it may become rather clear throughout, particularly in the next section, where I discuss risk balancing and the moral trade-offs and contradictions it necessarily involves, that I do not believe in such a thing).

36. MacIntyre, *After Virtue*, 64.

37. See, for example, Remington et al., "Increasing Food Acceptance"; Cooke et al., "Eating for Pleasure"; Fildes et al., "Randomized Controlled Trial." Note, however, that these studies all focus on modifying children's tastes and do not conclusively demonstrate significant long-term effects.

38. Singer, "'Why Can't You Be,'" 64.

39. Blume, "Neurodiversity." This was the first use of the term *neurodiversity* in print, though Singer coined it after conversations with Blume. Blume had

previously used the term *neurological pluralism* to describe a similar concept. Blume, "Autistics, Freed." For more on this exchange, see Silberman, *Neurotribes*, 450–56.

40. Quoted in Silberman, chap. 11, part IV, from pers. comm. between Silberman and Singer.

41. I am, all other things being equal, in favor of identity-first language (so "an autistic person" rather than "a person with autism"). However, I say "someone with ADHD" for the simple and perhaps petty reason that I can think of no way to turn the initialism "ADHD" into an adjective (like "autistic") that I don't find aesthetically appalling.

42. Groner, "Sex as 'Spock,'" 273.

43. Groner, 267.

44. Groner, 267.

45. For an argument about the moral implications of this claim, see, for example, Leach Scully, *Disability Bioethics*.

46. Buber, *I and Thou*.

47. Levinas, *Totality and Infinity*, 72.

48. Zoloth, *Healthcare and the Ethics*, 145. Here, Zoloth is reading Levinas through a distinctly practical lens.

49. Rubin, "Thinking Sex," 293.

50. Wendell, "Unhealthy Disabled."

51. Kafer, Feminist, Queer, Crip, 83.

3. Risky Business

1. McRuer, *Crip Theory*; Sandahl, "Queering the Crip."

2. Douglas and Wildavsky, *Risk and Culture*.

3. Kasperson et al., "Social Amplification of Risk."

4. Certainly the prevailing principlist model of biomedical ethics, classically articulated by Thomas Beauchamp and James F. Childress in *Principles of Biomedical Ethics*, can be understood in terms of risk balancing: providers must weigh the risks and benefits to each of the four key principles of autonomy, justice, beneficence, and nonmaleficence. A given course of action may pose a high level of danger to the patient's welfare (beneficence or nonmaleficence, depending on the particulars), but if the patient has clearly indicated they prefer that course of action, not doing so may pose significant danger to their autonomy. For examinations of risk perceptions in specific clinical contexts, see, for example, on risk perception in obstetrics, Minkoff and Marshall, "Fetal Risks, Relative Risks"; and Lyerly et al., "R I S K." On risk perception and informed consent, see, for example, Ankeny and Kerridge, "On Not Taking Objective."

5. Freedman, *Duty and Healing*, 320.

6. Welch, *Feminist Ethic of Risk*, 47.

7. Perske, "Dignity of Risk"; Wolpert, "Dignity of Risk." See also DeJong, "Independent Living"; Deegan, "Independent Living Movement."

8. See, for example, Mez et al., "Clinicopathological Evaluation." And see, for example, Ball et al., "Equestrian Injuries"; Paix, "Rider Injury Rates"; Bond, Christoph, and Rodgers, "Pediatric Equestrian Injuries"; Winkler et al., "Adult Sports-Related Traumatic."

9. McRuer, *Crip Theory*, 2.

10. McRuer, 7–8.

11. Sandhal, "Queering the Crip."

12. Perry and Carter-Long, "Ruderman White Paper."

13. McBryde Johnson, "Disability Gulag."

14. Mingus, "Forced Intimacy."

15. Zisk, "I Hid," 190.

16. Bascom, "Speech, Without a Title," 192.

17. Bascom, 195.

18. McRuer, *Crip Theory*, 10.

19. McRuer, 156; emphasis mine, except for emphasis on the word "likelihood," which is in the original.

20. McRuer, 156–57.

21. Mingus, "Access Intimacy."

22. Mingus.

23. Kafer, *Feminist, Queer, Crip*, 128.

24. Wendell, "Unhealthy Disabled."

25. Kafer, *Feminist, Queer, Crip*, 83. See also Eva Feder Kittay's "dependency critique" of liberal feminist accounts of autonomy, in *Love's Labor: Essays on Women, Equality, and Dependency*.

26. Mullin, *Reconceiving Pregnancy and Childcare*, 46.

27. The bio-psychosocial policing of pregnant and potentially pregnant people, and in particular the ways in which this policing is racialized, is a significant and incredibly important phenomenon to which this project lacks the scope to do justice. But see, to begin with, Kukla, *Mass Hysteria*, on the history and ethics of policing the "unruly" pregnant body; and Roberts, *Killing the Black Body*; as well as Cooper Owens, *Medical Bondage*, on the history of the development of American obstetrics and gynecology as a site of racial and gender oppression.

28. Centers for Disease Control and Prevention, "Burden of Foodborne Illness."

29. US Fire Administration, "U.S. Fire Statistics."

30. Fredrickson and Losada, "Positive Affect," 1.

31. Fredrickson and Losada, 10.

32. See, for example, Christopher Ryan and Cacilda Jetha's work of popular evolutionary psychology, *Sex at Dawn: How We Mate, Why We Stray, and What It*

Means for Modern Relationships. This book—whose central claim is that monogamy is unnatural for humans—received a significant amount of attention in some "sex-positive" circles. There has been some justified criticism of Ryan and Jetha's cherry-picking of anthropological and ethological data. Even aside from these factual challenges, the simplistic character of their argument—"hunter-gatherers were and are promiscuous; therefore, monogamy is unnatural, and socio-cultural enforcement of monogamy is harmful and immoral"—betrays a shallow grasp of the development of cultural values and the complexity of moral thought, particularly where religion is concerned. Sadly, this short-sightedness, particularly about religion, is not uncommon among modern and contemporary sexuality writers. Jesse Bering's otherwise fascinating book *Perv: The Sexual Deviant in All of Us* provides a paradigmatic example when he claims that "religious individuals point to Matthew 5:28" (22) when they talk about sex—something that would come as a bit of a surprise to a devout Jew, Muslim, or Hindu!

33. This is to say nothing of the fact that the term *natural* is frustratingly vague: Do we mean it in an Aristotelian sense as being the "substance of those things with a principle or process within themselves *qua* themselves"? Aristotle, *Metaphysics*, 1015b/119. Or do we mean it, as I do—and as I suspect many other writers on this topic would also—in a more Deweyan sense as being the sum of all phenomena, a dynamic "affair of affairs"? Dewey, *Experience and Nature*, 97. On this view, nature is a category that is potentially infinitely inclusive. To engage in practical moral judgment, however, is to necessarily engage in acts of differentiation and exclusion. Categories on which we base moral judgments, therefore, require clearer and more robust limiting principles than the category of natural can provide.

34. Dewey, 112.

35. For more on the ways people, especially multiply marginalized people, do, in fact, exercise wise sexual risk management, see, for example, Longmire-Avital, "'I Asked,'" a study of Black women's sexual risk negotiation strategies; Longmire-Avital and Oberle, "'Condoms are the Standard'"; Walker, Longmire-Avital, and Golub, "Racial and Sexual Identities"; and Golub et al., "Role of Religiosity."

36. Welch, *Feminist Ethic of Risk*, 68.

37. See, among others, Nussbaum, *Upheavals of Thought*; and Ahmed, *Cultural Politics of Emotion* and *Willful Subjects*.

38. Neis, *Sense of Sight*, 158–67. See Boyarin, *Carnal Israel* and *Unheroic Conduct*; and Neis.

39. Here, R. Yoḥanan is described as beardless, and his beauty is described as resembling a silver goblet filled with pomegranate arils and rose petals, caught in *just* the perfect light. Between this, and the description of him as notably fat in Berakhot 13b, personally speaking, I picture what you might describe as a gorgeously fat twink. Think Darienne Lake from season 6 of *Ru Paul's Drag Race*, out of drag.

40. Following Daniel Boyarin in *Carnal Israel* and *Unheroic Conduct*, my translation here takes the explicit details about Resh Laḳish thinking Rabbi Yoḥanan is a woman and vaulting the river on his lance from a manuscript variant, Hamburg 19.

41. For an extensive, if irreverent, catalog of instances of this trope in various popular media, see "Replacement Goldfish," *TV Tropes* (blog), accessed April 18, 2022, https://tvtropes.org/pmwiki/pmwiki.php/Main/ReplacementGoldfish.

42. Rubenstein, Culture of the Babylonian, 43.

Part II: Case Studies on Community and Risk

1. Magness, *Stone and Dung*; Miller, *At the Intersection*; Furstenberg, *Purity and Community*.

2. Halbertal, *Mahapekhot Parshaniyot Be-Hit'havutan*; Lorberbaum, "Tselem Elohim" and "Adam, Dam, Demut"; Steinmetz, "Crimes and Punishments, Part I" and "Crimes and Punishments, Part II"; Shemesh, *Punishments and Sins*.

3. Rosen-Zvi, *Mishnaic Sotah Ritual*; Ahuvia, "Analogies of Violence."

4. STIs

1. Most benignly, relatively speaking, the World Health Organization (WHO) estimates that 67 percent of adults under fifty worldwide have herpes simplex virus type 1 (HSV-1; primarily oral), and another 13 percent have HSV-2 (primarily genital). WHO, "Herpes Simplex Virus." More worrisome is the Centers for Disease Control and Prevention's (CDC) 2015 report, according to which total combined cases in the United States of chlamydia, gonorrhea, and primary and secondary syphilis—which were at historic lows for gonorrhea in 2009 and syphilis in 2000 and 2001—reached the highest rates yet measured. CDC, *Sexually Transmitted Disease Surveillance*, 1–2. Rates of all three infections increased between 2014 and 2015, with syphilis showing the most precipitous increase. Syphilis rates rose by 19 percent during this period. Additionally, rates of congenital syphilis (which occurs when someone who is pregnant passes a syphilis infection to the fetus) increased for the first time since 2008, by 27.2 percent in 2013–2014 and 6 percent in 2014–2015. CDC, 2. Gonorrhea rates also rose sharply—by 12.8 percent—since 2014, and antibiotic-resistant strains of gonorrhea are a serious and worsening problem. CDC, 1–2. Global STI rates are also increasing. In 2008, the WHO reported a total increase of 11.3 percent in combined cases of chlamydia, gonorrhea, syphilis, and *Trichomonas vaginalis* from 2005. The WHO also estimates that in 2013 there were 35 million people living with HIV/AIDS, of whom 1.5 million died that year of AIDS-related illnesses. The report also showed a 4.1 percent increase in chlamydia, a 21 percent increase in gonorrhea, an 11.2 percent increase in *Trichomonas vaginalis*, and a steady rate of syphilis infection. WHO, "Global Health Observatory Data."

2. In addition to morbidity and mortality that occur as a direct consequence of such infections as untreated syphilis or HIV, STIs can have serious secondary complications, including several kinds of cancers and such complications as pelvic inflammatory disease, ectopic pregnancy, epididymitis, prostatitis, and infertility. STIs can cause pregnancy complications and can be transmitted from mother to infant, leading in turn to a host of congenital problems for the newborn. See Eng and Butler, *Hidden Epidemic*, 46, table 2–3, for a more comprehensive list of sequelae. STIs can also facilitate the transmission of other STIs, compounding the problem—for example, an active herpes infection can facilitate the transmission of HIV. Eng and Butler, 49–56.

3. Several highly effective technical and behavioral interventions exist; they become even more effective when combined. Vaccines for hepatitis A and B have been in use since 1995 and 1982 respectively. A vaccine for the four strains of HPV most linked to cancers and genital warts has been available since 2006; a new formulation that prevents five additional strains of HPV was approved by the FDA in 2014. External and internal condoms, used regularly and correctly, are highly effective at preventing the spread of fluid-transmitted infections and reduce the risk of infections transmitted by skin-to-skin contact. CDC, "Condoms and STDs." Pre-exposure prophylaxis (PrEP), when used consistently and in combination with regular testing, is up to 92 percent effective in stopping the transmission of HIV. CDC, "Pre-Exposure Prophylaxis (PrEP)." And an HIV-positive individual whose viral load is undetectable can become practically noninfectious. See, for example, Schader and Wainberg, "Insights into HIV-1 Pathogenesis," 91–98. Suppressive therapy can also reduce the transmission risk from a person who has HSV-1 or HSV-2. CDC, "2015 Sexually Transmitted Diseases." Behavioral interventions also work. At the individual level, clinician counseling, couple-based interventions, and workshops (especially those guided by cognitive-behavioral theory) aimed at practicing the sorts of interpersonal skills necessary to alter sexual behavior all seem to precipitate significant changes, at least in the short term. Institute of Medicine (IOM), *Hidden Epidemic*, 134–35. Condom distribution programs in schools and other institutions also appear to significantly increase condom use. See, for example, Charania et al., "Efficacy of Structural-Level," 1293. This meta-analysis concluded that structural-level interventions that "increased the availability of condoms, or increased accessibility to condoms, as a distribution strategy were efficacious in increasing condom use behaviors." Such programs were effective among diverse populations and became even more effective when combined with "additional individual, small group, or community-level activities." At the community level, effective interventions often address structural and environmental conditions that might be barriers to behavior change and focus on high-risk groups and position individuals from within those high-risk groups as educators, mentors, and role models. Charania et al., 137. In other words, effective behavioral

interventions seem to teach people what to do sexually rather than merely focusing on what not to do. Particularly effective ways of teaching people what to do include practicing positive behaviors and providing exemplars and role models for those behaviors—results that should not surprise virtue ethicists!

4. See, for example, Luo et al., "Optimal Antiviral Switching."

5. People with vaginas, uteri, and ovaries, for example, tend to be affected far more seriously by the complications of STIs than people with penises, for a number of reasons. Being penetrated—though it is important to note that those with internal genitals do not always assume the sexual role of the penetrated, nor do those with external genitals always assume the role of the penetrator—exposes one to greater risk of transmission than does penetrating someone. Furthermore, STIs are harder to detect and more likely to remain asymptomatic in internal reproductive tracts for a longer period, delaying diagnosis and treatment as well. See IOM, *Hidden Epidemic*, 35. Sexual abuse is another route of STI transmission that is outside the victim's control. IOM, 79–80. The IOM further notes (75) that those populations with the poorest access to health services are the same populations that have the highest STI rates. Insurance coverage for STI screening services can be spotty, and the availability of funding and staff for community clinics that are likely to serve marginalized populations remains tenuous. This is especially true in a political climate that seeks to restrict access to reproductive health clinics. Such restriction occurs most visibly in the name of antiabortion activism, but it also has to do with antipoverty and antisex stigma, as well as opposition to contraception. Even assuming access to regular clinical care, rates of routine STI screening in primary care settings remain well below recommended levels. IOM, 95; St. Lawrence et al., "STI Screening, Testing"; Cook et al., "Barriers to Screening"; Millstein, Igra, and Gans, "Delivery of STD/HIV." Furthermore, people in economically tenuous situations may, quite understandably, give lower priority to reproductive health care than to more immediate concerns: "Even if a person in poverty perceives himself or herself to be at risk for an STD, he or she may not practice preventive behaviors if there are other risks that appear more imminent or more threatening or both." IOM, 75. Racial and economic minorities bear a greater STI burden, mainly due to disparities in access to health care and social services of any kind. For US data, see CDC, *Sexually Transmitted Disease Surveillance*, 2, 69–76. For global data, see WHO, *Global Incidence and Prevalence*; WHO, "Global Health Observatory Data"; Joint United Nations Programme on HIV/AIDS, *Global Report*, 12; UNAIDS "Fact Sheet"; Joint United Nations Programme on HIV/AIDS, *Gap Report 2014*. Importantly, these disparities cannot be explained by divergent sexual risk behavior: for example, African Americans, who have higher rates of a number of STIs than whites, also use condoms at notably higher rates than do whites: "African American women are almost twice as likely to use condoms compared to women of other races. In addition, African American men are more likely to have used condoms during their last

episode of intercourse compared to either European American or Hispanic men."
IOM, 148. But structurally oppressed communities also face social barriers to sexual
and reproductive health care because STIs have historically been associated with
minority groups such that persistent conditions of sexually transmitted disease are
assumed to be these groups' natural state. Even when these groups have had access
to care, they have often been treated unequally or even actively harmed, as in the
case of the infamous Tuskegee study (the classic treatment of which is James H.
Jones's *Bad Blood: The Tuskegee Syphilis Experiment*) but hardly limited to that. See,
for example, Washington, *Medical Apartheid*; and Cooper Owens, *Medical Bondage*.

6. Juvenal's second satire, for example, mentions anal warts and links them to
an overindulgence in receptive anal intercourse. See Oriel, *Scars of Venus*, 155.

7. See Quetel, *History of Syphilis*, 22–23.

8. Gilino of Ferrera, *De Morbo quem gallicum nuncupant*, quoted in Parascandola, *Sex, Sin, and Science*, 3.

9. Gilman, *Jew's Body*, 96; Parascandola, 4–5; Quetel, *History of Syphilis*, 33.

10. As Parascandola puts it, "The Italians called syphilis the French disease,
while the French called it the Neapolitan disease. The Japanese blamed the Chi-
nese, the Russians the Poles, and the Persians the Turks for the spread of the pox.
Placing the blame on American Indians removed the stigma from Europe entirely,
assigning responsibility to an external 'Other' (the Indian)." Parascandola, 5.

11. Quetel, *History of Syphilis*, 22–23. In the same year the town council of Ab-
erdeen, in Scotland, "ordered all 'loose women' to desist from 'the sins of venery.'"
Quetel, 8.

12. See P. Levine, *Prostitution, Race, and Politics*; and Gilman, *Jew's Body*. Interestingly, in the nineteenth and early twentieth centuries, there existed a dual
picture in which syphilis was figured as a Jewish disease while, at the same time,
Jews were often painted as being immune to syphilis. This supposed immunity
was often linked to the practice of circumcision, but not always—there was also
speculation about the Jew being constitutionally immune to syphilis as well. See
Gilman, as well as Hart, *Healthy Jew*; and Presner, *Muscular Judaism*.

13. Parascandola describes several propaganda posters from this era, noting
of posters aimed at enlisted men during World War II that, "when personified,
venereal disease was always portrayed as a woman in these posters, [for example, a
poster featuring a] female figure with the face of death marching arm-in-arm with
Hitler and Tojo." This poster bears the caption "VD: Worst of the Three." Parascandola, *Sex, Sin, and Science*, 116. Several of these posters are available for viewing at
the National Library of Medicine. National Library of Medicine, "Visual Culture."

14. Quoted in Vonlehrer and Heller, "New Attack on Venereal Disease."

15. Godwin added that he was "upset that the Government is not spending
more money to protect the general public from the gay plague." Clendinen, "AIDS
Spreads Pain." Also quoted in Brandt, *No Magic Bullet*, 183.

16. Smith et al., "Effects of Human Papillomavirus."

17. As Brandt notes: "In 1908 the Massachusetts Association of Boards of Health published a circular for young women, warning them of the consequences of premarital sex. 'Among the most serious dangers which threaten young women, especially those of the wage-earning class,' noted the pamphlet, 'is the danger of sexual relations outside of marriage to which they are led by such harmless pleasures as dancing.'" Brandt, *No Magic Bullet*, 26.

18. Brandt, 31–32.

19. Brandt, 32. The term was coined by Prince Morrow of the American Society for Sanitary and Moral Prophylaxis.

20. IOM, *Hidden Epidemic*, 90. As the report notes, "Conversations regarding healthy sexual behaviors and STDs do not take place when parents deny that their children are sexually active or that adolescents have sexual drives. . . . Because many parents do not talk about sex with their children, children are more likely to learn about sex through clandestine and secretive exchanges with peers that result in a massive amount of misinformation."

21. IOM, 91.

22. IOM, 95.

23. IOM, 99. Failing to speak openly and accurately about STIs also means that they are often treated as a single category, with the consequence that some STIs are ignored. HIV, for example, has in the past few decades become the paradigmatic STI—understandably so, since it is almost certainly fatal if untreated. Between the advent of effective antiretroviral drugs that have changed HIV from a certain death sentence to a chronic, survivable condition and the recent advent of PrEP drugs, HIV/AIDS has become less threatening. Yet the defanging of HIV/AIDS (in the affluent West, at least) does not eliminate the threat of other STIs—for example, frightening new strains of antibiotic-resistant gonorrhea. This would not be the first time gonorrhea in particular has been overlooked in favor of other infections: Brandt notes that during the New Deal–era antisyphilis campaigns, "while massive testing for syphilis was undertaken in the 1930s, little interest in the other major venereal disease, gonorrhea, was expressed by public health officials. . . . Syphilis made headlines, while gonorrhea, four times more prevalent than syphilis, receded deeper into the public consciousness." Brandt, *No Magic Bullet*, 154.

24. Balberg classifies these practices according to two categories: "examination of the day," which is "an ongoing effort to give oneself an account of all one's activities and encounters that could have exposed one or one's possessions to impurity," and "self-examination of the body," in which one searches for "signs that will attest to a bodily state that renders one impure"—impure genital discharges, for example, or impure lesions of the skin. Balberg, *Purity, Body, and Self*, 157.

25. The first line of M. Niddah 2:1 appears to complicate this claim: "Every hand that examines frequently—in women, it is praiseworthy, but in men, it should be

cut off." The line, which refers specifically to the examination of genital discharges and which is classically interpreted as discouraging masturbation in men, is certainly a problematic one, as it simultaneously discourages men from one potentially valuable mode of self-knowledge and places a disproportionate burden of examination on women (although it is possible to put forth a counterinterpretation in which it figures *women* as the paradigmatic self-examiners).

Nevertheless, for my purposes here, I do not believe the passage disproves my claim that self-examination, writ large, is virtuous for *everyone*. M. Niddah 2:1 discourages men from engaging in one specific form of self-examination of the genitals—it states that the hand that examines frequently in men ought to be cut off. It does not discourage men from examining the body (including the genitals) more generally, nor does it discourage them from examining their memories of the day. Indeed, much of the language in Zavim refers literally to *seeing* episodes of discharge, suggesting that visual examination of the genitals is still encouraged, even if tactile examination is not.

26. Balberg, *Purity, Body, and Self*, 148–79. See, for example, p. 164: "[Mishnaic] practices [of self-examination both assume and generate] *a subject distinguished by his self-command and self-consciousness. . . . Self-examination is also self-formation*" (emphasis in the original).

27. See, for example, Gottlieb et al., "Toward Global Prevention"; and Mabey, "Epidemiology." Both articles specifically note the asymptomatic character of many STIs as a factor in their transmission.

28. The sex advice columnist Dan Savage has had to remind numerous callers who are afraid of continuing a relationship with a partner who has disclosed that they are HIV positive that one may be at greater risk of infection from someone who (wrongly) assumes or (falsely) claims they are HIV negative than someone with a known and well-managed HIV infection. See, for example, Savage, "Magnum Episode #365," where Savage responds to a caller who is in the early stages of a relationship with someone who has just disclosed their HIV-positive status:

> A huge percentage of people who are positive don't know they're positive. There are many people out there running around who think they're HIV-negative, may have been negative the last time they got an HIV test, who are now HIV-positive. And paradoxically, you are at more risk being in a sexual relationship with someone who thinks he's negative and isn't, than you are in a relationship with someone who knows he's positive and is under treatment. Most people who are positive and are being treated have zero viral load. They are—doctors will say they are functionally non-infectious. They pose, really, no threat. If you're also then not having anal intercourse, you're not doing anything that puts you at greater risk for HIV transmission, if he *were* crazy infectious or if his viral load is for some reason spiking because his meds are off, you're really at very, very little risk.

Savage's claim about risk seems supported by the results of HIV Prevention Trial Network, "HPTN 052," which showed a 93 percent reduction in HIV transmission among serodiscordant couples in which the HIV-positive partner received early antiretroviral treatment. Notably, out of 1,171 couples in both treatment arms (so both early and delayed antiretroviral treatment) who completed the study, only eight cases of transmission were reported after the HIV-positive partner began treatment.

29. Ritual impurity is fairly easy to contract and relatively easy to remedy. It is temporary, mainly comes from contact with bodies of some kind, and is etiologically unrelated to sin. Moral impurity, conversely, arises as the direct result of committing a sin. Ritual impurity is individually contracted, is shared only when the contractor comes into certain defined types of contact with others, and is an immediate problem only in the sanctuary. Moral impurity affects the entire community, regardless of who within the community committed the sin. Ritual impurity's effects are immediate, limited, and temporary. Moral impurity's effects are often delayed, usually permanent, and cumulative, polluting the community, land, and sancta over time. This concept was worked out variously by David Zvi Hoffman, Jacob Milgrom, and Tikva Frymer-Kensky and then further developed by Jonathan Klawans. See Hoffman, *Das Buch Leviticus*; Milgrom, "Sin-Offering or Purification-Offering?" and *Leviticus 1–16*; Frymer-Kensky, "Pollution, Purification, and Purgation"; and Klawans, *Impurity and Sin*.

30. See Balberg, *Purity, Body, and Self*, several places, including 28, 35.

31. I'm grateful to Elizabeth Shanks Alexander (personal correspondence, August 20, 2021) for encouraging me to make this point explicit and framing it so clearly in the terms I use here.

32. Although certain persons, like the amei ha'arets, are assumed to be default carriers of impurity, this is not because it is a more "native" status for them and alien to others but rather because the amei ha'arets are assumed to take insufficient care regarding the default impurity with which the entire community must deal. Further, the exclusion of Gentiles from the purity system complicates the claim that impurity is "everyone's problem." Gentiles, prior to conversion, cannot contract impurity, although they can transmit it. They do not fully participate in the economy of purity, impurity, and sacred space that makes a pure or impure status relevant. This exclusion strains the parallel with STIs as far as universality is concerned. STIs are a risk for everyone, in every community; they exist and have measurable health consequences regardless of whether they are religiously or culturally relevant to their victims and vectors. However, as a model for how we understand STI risk as a social phenomenon, the fact that the very ability to contract impurity indicates a privileged status is instructive and even corrective. If impurity is an unavoidable consequence of certain kinds of social relations, it follows that someone who can fully participate in the purity economy is someone

who engages in those social relations. And, although the partial exclusion of Gentiles from this economy has problematic implications about who is in and who is out of a privileged group, it is important to note that within purity discourse, it is the more privileged classes that can contract impurity. STIs have historically been treated as diseases of the Other. But impurity is not the default condition of the Other; if anything, a lack of full participation in the system of impurity is a marker of Otherness. Entering a social context in which purity becomes a relevant, applicable risk is, all in all, a praiseworthy and esteemed action. The relationships that make impurity relevant are worthwhile in and of themselves. Balberg, *Purity, Body, and Self,* 28.

33. See Balberg's discussion (153) of the amei ha'arets, "people of the land," a group whose identity is the subject of some debate but who at the very least can be understood as Jews looked down upon by the rabbis, are primarily identified within the Mishnah by "their notable carelessness regarding impurity, at least according to rabbinic standards." The amei ha'arets are assumed to be perpetually impure, not because they cannot become pure by virtue of existing outside the rabbinic system (like Gentiles) but because of "their insufficient efforts to maintain a state of purity in their everyday lives." Interestingly, though the carelessness of the amei ha'arets occasions disdain, it does not occasion shunning: the texts assume that anything handled by an am ha'arets is impure, but they also assume one will have at least semiregular interactions with amei ha'arets. Balberg, 153. For more on the relationship between impurity and the particulars of in-group versus out-group membership, see Hayes, *Gentile Impurities.*

34. Looker et al., "Global and Regional Estimates"; Looker et al., "Global Estimates."

35. See, for example, Planned Parenthood, "Safer Sex ('Safe Sex')"; and Pierce, "What Is Safer Sex."

36. Balberg, *Purity, Body, and Self,* 145.

37. Wald and Corey, "Persistence in the Population." CDC, "Genital Herpes."

38. In fact, the actual rate is probably even higher since an infected individual may never experience symptoms or may fail to recognize them as evidence of a herpes infection.

39. M. Kelim 1:4; M. Kelim 1:3.

40. M. Kelim 1:3.

41. M. Kelim 1:5.

42. M. Kelim 1:4; M. Kelim 1:1.

43. This is an example of what Balberg refers to as a broader "graded system of impurity," in which the initial source, referred to as the "father" of impurity, has the strongest power to transmit. Someone or something the "father" of impurity touches becomes a "first" of impurity, who has diminished power to transmit; someone or something the "first" touches is a "second" of impurity, with even

further diminished power; and so on. So in this case, the zav is the father of impurity, what he lies on is a first, a person who touches what he lies on is a second, and so on. Balberg, *Purity, Body, and Self*, 28–30.

44. This is an example of transmission by "shift" (*heset*). There are other modes of transmission by indirect contact: "treading" or "leaning" (*midras*), for example, is invoked in a case where a zav and someone who is pure sit together on a boat or ride an animal together, even though they are not physically touching in either circumstance. See M. Zavim 3:1.

45. See, for example, Schader and Wainberg, "Insights into HIV-1 Pathogenesis," 91–98.

46. See McElligott, "Mortality from Sexually Transmitted."

47. This is not to say that drug resistance does not also affect HIV: it does, especially when patients fail to take their antiretroviral drugs regularly. It is to say, however, that antibiotic resistance seems to be a much more widespread and rapidly developing problem for the treatment of gonorrhea.

48. I use the term *hyperfocus*, which, clinically speaking, refers to the way people with ADHD focus on a desired subject or activity for hours on end, deliberately. See chap. 2.

49. Balberg, Purity, Body, and Self, 28.

5. BDSM

1. Berkowitz, *Execution and Invention*, 163.

2. Weiss, *Techniques of Pleasure*, 24.

3. See Musser, *Sensational Flesh*, 44.

4. Rubinstein, *Culture of the Babylonian*, 57–58, referring to b. Rosh Hashana 13a and b. Sanhedrin 30b, b. Pesachim 69a, and b. Yevamot 106a, respectively.

5. Rubenstein, 57–58.

6. Schofer, *Making of a Sage*, 72. Schofer notes that the compilers of Avot D'Rabbi Natan were especially wary of four passages in the Solomonic tradition—Song of Songs 7:11–13, Ecclesiastes 11:9, and Proverbs 7—which they considered either too erotic or, in the case of Ecclesiastes, far too sanguine about the integrity of any individual's judgment. Schofer, 73.

7. Schofer, 76. For example, Rabbi Natan 1:5 reads the difference between Genesis 2:17 (in which God instructs Adam not to eat of the tree of knowledge lest he die) and Genesis 3:3 (in which Eve informs the serpent that they may not touch the tree lest they die) as Adam's attempt to create a fence for Eve around God's initial instruction. Yet "Adam's version of the law is vulnerable to falsification." The serpent touches the tree and is not struck dead, and so Eve doubts the veracity of everything else Adam, "her rabbi," has taught her.

8. Schofer, 76.

9. Schofer, 76.

10. See, for example, Rubenstein's treatment of b. Bava Kamma 117a.

11. Rubenstein, *Culture of the Baylonian*, 51.

12. Rubenstein, 59.

13. Schofer, *Making of a Sage*, 95.

14. As Schofer writes of a forge as a metaphor for the discipline of the self in Avot D'Rabbi Natan A16:64, "when immersed in the flames of Torah, the [bad yetser's] tendencies and energies become useful. . . . Torah [is] a transformative force that is far more powerful than the yetser or the heart." Schofer, 96.

15. It is suggestive that the text immediately employs ophidian imagery, and it is especially suggestive that it is the argumentative activity of the sages themselves that is compared to a snake. In other rabbinic texts, snakes (there are several words used for them) often represent risk or danger: Bavli Berakhot 33a, for example, discusses whether a snake curled at one's heel is sufficiently dangerous to interrupt one's prayer, and Berakhot 62a mentions snakes as one of the three dangers modest bathroom habits protect against. Snakes also appear as guardians of tombs; indeed, when in Bava Metzia 84b and Bava Kama 117b the specific word for snake used here, *akhan*, occurs, it identifies a snake coiled with its tail in its mouth at the entrance to a sage's tomb. Also cf. Mira Wasserman's discussion of snakes and gentiles in Bavli Avodah Zara in her recent *Jews, Gentiles, and Other Animals*.

16. Cubits; roughly, arms-lengths.

17. Newmahr, *Playing on the Edge*, 75.

18. Switch, "Origin of RACK."

19. Other important terms include *play*, which can refer to the general practice of BDSM or to specific instances of it (although through the 1980s or so it was also common to use *work* in a similar sense). A *scene* refers to any discrete instances of BDSM play involving two or more people; it can also refer to the BDSM community or BDSM culture at large, for example, "the Bay Area scene." Within a scene, a *top* is a person who is acting upon a relatively passive *bottom*; a *switch* may change roles. *Top, bottom*, and *switch* are also markers of identity; within the broader BDSM scene (rather than *a* scene), a person may prefer to play the role of and be known as one of these terms. For more detailed definitions of key terms, see, for example, Taormino, "'S is for . . .'," 3–32.

20. Newmahr, *Playing on the Edge*, 84.

21. Weiss, *Techniques of Pleasure*, 12.

22. Weiss, 12.

23. Weiss, 87.

24. Newmahr, *Playing on the Edge*, 78.

25. Newmahr, 80.

26. Newmahr, 84.

27. Newmahr, 87.

28. Newmahr, 88.

29. Newmahr, 88–89.

30. See Wiseman, *SM 101*, 58–62, for an example. Weiss, *Techniques of Pleasure*, 81. See also Wiseman, 58–62; Newmahr, *Playing on the Edge*, 75–78; Scott, *Thinking Kink*, 88–96, Taormino, "S is for . . .'"; and Johanns, "Channels of Cum-munica-tion," 5–12, among others, for more on negotiation and safe words.

31. Johanns, 6–7.

32. Weiss, *Techniques of Pleasure*, 83.

33. Chow, "Politics of Admittance," 64.

34. Sisson, "Cultural Formation of S/M," 19.

35. Sisson, 28.

36. Newmahr, *Playing on the Edge*, 25–38.

37. Schofer, *Making of a Sage*, ch. 2.

38. Newmahr, *Playing on the Edge*, ch. 2.

39. Weiss, *Techniques of Pleasure*, 56.

40. Weiss, 57 (emphasis mine).

41. Weiss, 122.

42. Weiss, 122.

43. Weiss, 122.

44. See, classically, the volume *Against Sadomasochism*. Indeed, this condemnation is founded on a version of the same claim that is foundational to this book: that sexual practice is a social relation that is inextricable from other social relations.

45. Weiss, *Techniques of Pleasure*, 150. See Hopkins, "Rethinking Sadomasochism"; Bateson, "Theory of Play"; Bauer, "Transgressive and Transformative." It is worth noting here that the extent to which BDSM practitioners understand what they do as play is one key point of tension between the "old guard" and the "new guard." Old-guard figures lament the current scene's apparent consumerism, as well as what they see as an overformality verging on legalism and a simultaneous trivialization of the practice. For example, in 2002, david stein, part of the committee who coined the integral terminology "safe, sane, and consensual" (SSC) wrote an essay in which he lamented the tokenization of the phrase: "The idolization of SSC occurred during the same period that S/M activity came to be almost universally referred to as play"—previously it was just as common to refer to it as work—"S/M practitioners as 'players,' and the tools we use as 'toys.'" stein "Safe, Sane, Consensual." Similarly, Gayle Rubin, even as she problematized the binary of "old guard/new guard," nevertheless lamented that "SM too often became a mechanical exercise rather than an art form or a form of intimate communication." Rubin, "Old Guard, New Guard." Such ambivalence continues into the present as BDSM culture and practice become further intertwined with technology, technocracy, and social media.

46. See, for example, Bauer; MacKendrick, *Counterpleasures*; McClintock, "Maid to Order."

47. See Berlant and Warner, "Sex in Public"; Esteban Muñoz, *Disidentifications*; Martin, "Extraordinary Homosexuals."

48. Weiss, *Techniques of Pleasure*, 160.

49. Weiss, 161.

50. Weiss, 182–83.

51. Weiss, 183.

52. Berkowitz, *Execution and Invention*, 154. See Bhaba, *Location of Culture*; and J. Scott, *Domination and the Arts*.

53. Berkowitz, 154.

54. Berkowitz, 160.

55. Berkowitz, 160. See Sifre Zuta 12, M. Nedarim 9:10, Sifra Behukotai 3:8.

56. Berkowitz, 160–61. See Sifre Deuteronomy 221 for the other use of the verbatim phrase, and see baraitot in b. Ketubot 30a, b. Sotah 8b, b. Sanhedrin 37b and 56a, b. Berakhot 32b, and b. Avodah Zarah 41, as well as Leviticus Rabbah 6:5 for sword symbolism and for decapitation as a Roman practice.

57. Berkowitz, 162. See Garnsey, "Why Penal Laws," 147; and Wiedemann, *Emperors and Gladiators*, 69.

58. Berkowitz, 163.

59. In 9:3 in most online editions.

60. Berkowitz, *Execution and Invention*, 163–64.

61. Berkowitz, 165.

62. Berkowitz, 165.

63. Lev. 20:2, 20:22, 24:14; Num. 15:34; Deut. 13:10, 21:21, 22:21. See Berkowitz, 107–8. "The stoning house was the height of two men. One of the witnesses pushes [the condemned] onto his loins. If he is turned on his heart, they turn him onto his loins. If he dies from this, [the court] has fulfilled [its obligation]. If not, the second [witness] picks up the stone and puts it onto his heart. And if he dies from this, it has fulfilled. If not, he is pelted with stones by all of Israel, as it is stated: 'The hand of the witnesses shall be first upon him to execute him, and the hand of all the people after'" (Deut. 17:7).

64. Berkowitz, 109. At the same time, later on in the tractate (m. Sanh. 11), the community's role as "audience to the collective spectacle of execution" (110) is greatly expanded, at least according to R. Akiva's opinion: R. Akiva holds that the execution of a rebellious elder should occur during a pilgrimage festival so that the whole community can be in attendance. His interlocutor, R. Judah, holds that the execution should occur immediately following a guilty verdict and that news of it should be sent everywhere. The parallel toseftas go even further than the Mishnah does, eliminating the community's understudy role in completing the stoning entirely (T. Sanh 9:6) while expanding the number of executions R. Akiva holds

should happen during a festival so that the whole of Israel may witness them (T. Sanh. 11:7). Thus, as Berkowitz notes, both biblical and rabbinic sources display "an inversely proportional relationship between agency and audience. . . . Leviticus and Deuteronomy express maximal agency for the community and a minimal role for the audience; the Mishnah minimizes agency and begins to emphasize audience" (111).

65. M. Sanhedrin 3:3–4, 4, 5. See Berkowitz, 120–21.

66. Deut 1:17: "Let the hands of the witnesses be the first against him to put him to death." While there is, as usual, a rabbinic disagreement as to just what this means, each interpretation is detailed and specific, leaving little room for individual discretion.

See, for ex., M. Sanh 6:4 and ms. variants, and T. Sanh. 9:6.

67. Berkowitz, *Execution and Invention*, 122 (emphasis mine).

68. Weiss, *Techniques of Pleasure*, 7.

69. Weiss, 160, 156.

70. Weiss, 158.

71. Weiss, 159.

72. See, classically, Cohen, *From the Maccabees*, 210–16. In the Middle Ages, however, there do seem to have been exceptions to this rule of rabbinic powerlessness regarding criminal judgment and punishment. See Farber, "Extra-Legal Punishments."

73. Indeed, more than one text draws a moral dichotomy between the bet midrash and the arena; Y. Berakhot 4:2, for example, thanks God, who "has given my portion among those who sit in the bet midrash and the synagogues, and has not given my portion to those in the theaters and the circuses. For I labor and they labor; I am conscientious and they are conscientious—but I labor to inherit the Garden of Eden, and they labor for the lowest pit." Yet, as Berkowitz points out, the rabbis create an unavoidable analogy between the bet midrash and the arena precisely by creating an extended rhetorical opposition: "Both the Rabbi and the Roman labor, but in different places and for different ends. . . . The Rabbis pair the study house with the theater in order to show the study house's superiority, but in the process they inextricably link the two." Berkowitz, *Execution and Invention*, 158.

74. Berkowitz, 71.

75. Weiss, *Techniques of Pleasure*, 219.

76. Cruz, *Color of Kink*, 50.

77. Williams is also one of Weiss's informants. Williams, "BDSM and Playing," 70.

78. Cruz, *Color of Kink*, 59; within this quoting Weiss, 205–6. See also Nash, *Black Body in Ecstasy*, for a similar analysis of the politics of Black women's participation in and consumption of pornography.

79. Musser, *Sensational Flesh*, 177.

80. Flanagan and Rose, *Pain Journal*, 112.

81. Flanagan and Rose, 44.

82. See Musser, *Sensational Flesh*, 128–33, for a fuller analysis of the juxtaposition of these two kinds of pain based, in part, on these particular journal entries.

83. Musser, 125.

84. As McRuer argues, in witnessing Flanagan's performances, "'some future person' or collectivity might detect in that sick message the seemingly incomprehensible way to survive, and survive well, at the margins of time, space, and representation they might, in fact, detect that surviving well can paradoxically mean surviving sick." McRuer, *Crip Theory*, 183. "Some future person" refers to Richard Kim's essay "Fuck the Future?," an unpublished essay quoted in the review essay Duggan, "Down There," 385–86.

85. Mekhilta D'Rabbi Ishmael, Masekhta de-ba Hodesh, Parshat Yitro 6.

86. Berkowitz, *Execution and Invention*, 159.

87. Indeed, by a later, Amoraic redaction of this sequence (Lev. Rabbah 24:14, parsha 32), the series of punishments has become wholly rabbinic: crucifixion no longer figures.

88. Berkowitz, *Execution and Invention*, 177.

89. Berkowitz, 176.

90. Berkowitz, 178.

91. Berkowitz, 179.

Conclusion

1. Note: the word for "wife" used here, *dvet'ho* (as opposed to *ishto*, "his woman") literally means "of his house."

2. Something the Bavli discusses explicitly in Shabbat 152b, where R. Shimon ben Ḥalafta laments that the "maker of peace in the home" has gone idle.

3. Jastrow, *A Dictionary of the Targumim*, 270–71.

4. Labovitz, "Heruta's Ruse," in Ruttenberg, *Passionate Torah*, 238.

5. Jastrow, 500.

6. The particular term used here for "inside it," *bagviah*, also has the (rare) valence of "penis," as in, for example, Ḳidushin 25a, which refers to an injury to *rosh hagviah*, "the extremity of the penis," as one of the blemishes on account of which a slave must be manumitted.

7. Sedgewick, *Epistemology of the Closet*, 5.

8. Califia, *Macho Sluts*, 58.

BIBLIOGRAPHY

Adler, Rachel. *Engendering Judaism: An Inclusive Theology and Ethics*. Boston: Beacon, 1998.

Ahmed, Sara. *The Cultural Politics of Emotion*. 2nd ed. Edinburgh: Edinburgh University Press, 2014.

———. *Willful Subjects*. Durham, NC: Duke University Press, 2014.

Ahuvia, Mika. "Analogies of Violence in Rabbinic Literature." *Journal of Feminist Studies in Religion* 34, no. 2 (Fall 2018): 59–74.

Ankeny, Rachel A., and Ian Kerridge. "On Not Taking Objective Risk Assessments at Face Value." *American Journal of Bioethics* 4, no. 3 (2004): 35–37. https://doi.org/10.1080/15265160490496750.

Aristotle. *Metaphysics*. Translated by Hugh Lawson-Tancred. London: Penguin, 1998.

Bal, Mieke. *Lethal Love: Feminist Literary Readings of Biblical Love Stories*. Bloomington: Indiana University Press, 1987.

Balberg, Mira. *Purity, Body, and Self in Ancient Rabbinic Literature*. Chicago: University of Chicago Press, 2014.

Ball, Chad G., Jill E. Ball, Andrew W. Kirkpatrick, and Robert H. Mulloy. "Equestrian Injuries: Incidence, Injury Patterns, and Risk Factors for 10 Years of Major Traumatic Injuries." *American Journal of Surgery* 193 (2007): 636–40. https://doi.org/10.1016/j.amjsurg.2007.01.016.

Bascom, Julia, ed. *Loud Hands: Autistic People, Speaking*. Washington, DC: Autistic Press, 2012.

———. "Speech, without a Title." In *Loud Hands: Autistic People, Speaking*, edited by Julia Bascom, 192–97. Washington, DC: Autistic Press, 2012.

Bateson, Gregory. "A Theory of Play and Fantasy." *Psychiatric Research Reports* 2 (1955): 39–51.

Bauer, Robin. "Transgressive and Transformative Gendered Sexual Practices and White Privileges: The Case of the Dyke/Trans BDSM Communities." *Women's Studies Quarterly* 36, no. 3/4 (2008): 233–53.

Beauchamp, Thomas, and James F. Childress. *Principles of Biomedical Ethics*. 7th ed. Oxford: Oxford University Press, 2012.

Bering, Jesse. *Perv: The Sexual Deviant in All of Us*. New York: Farrar, Straus, and Giroux, 2013.

Berkovits, Eliezer. "A Jewish Sexual Ethics." In *Essential Essays on Judaism*, edited by David Hazony, 103–28. Jerusalem: Shalem, 2002.

Berkowitz, Beth A. *Execution and Invention: Death Penalty Discourse in Early Rabbinic and Christian Cultures*. Oxford: Oxford University Press, 2006.

Berlant, Lauren, and Michael Warner. "Sex in Public." *Critical Inquiry* 24, no. 2 (1998): 547–66.

Bhaba, Homi K. *The Location of Culture*. London: Routledge, 1994.

Blume, Harvey. "Autistics, Freed from Face-to-Face Encounters, Are Communicating in Cyberspace." *New York Times*, June 30, 1997. https://www.nytimes .com/1997/06/30/business/autistics-freed-from-face-to-face-encounters-are -communicating-in-cyberspace.html.

———. "Neurodiversity: On the Neurological Underpinnings of Geekdom." *The Atlantic*, September 1998. https://www.theatlantic.com/magazine/archive /1998/09/neurodiversity/305909/.

Bond, G. R., R. A. Christoph, and B. M. Rodgers. "Pediatric Equestrian Injuries: Assessing the Impact of Helmet Use." *Pediatrics* 95, no. 4 (April 1995): 487–89.

Borowitz, Eugene B. *Choosing a Sex Ethic: A Jewish Inquiry*. New York: Schocken Books, 1969.

Boyarin, Daniel. *Carnal Israel: Reading Sex in Talmudic Culture*. Berkeley: University of California Press, 1993.

———. *Socrates and the Fat Rabbis*. Chicago: University of Chicago Press, 2009.

———. *Unheroic Conduct: The Rise of Heterosexuality and the Invention of the Jewish Man*. Berkeley: University of California Press, 1997.

Brandt, Allan M. *No Magic Bullet: A Social History of Venereal Disease in the United States Since 1880*. New York: Oxford University Press, 1985.

Brown, Peter. *The Body and Society: Men, Women, and Sexual Renunciation in Early Christianity*. New York: Columbia University Press, 1988.

Brown Douglas, Kelly. "Black and Blues: God Talk / Body Talk for the Black Church." In *Womanist Theological Ethics: A Reader*, edited by Katie Geneva

Cannon, Emilie M. Townes, and Angela D. Sims, 127–28. Louisville, KY: Westminster John Knox Press, 2011.

———. *Sexuality and the Black Church: A Womanist Perspective.* New York: Orbis Books, 1999.

Broyde, Michael J. "The Foundations of Law: A Jewish Law View of World Law." *Emory Law Journal* 54, no. 3 (2005): 79–80.

Buber, Martin. *I and Thou.* Translated by Walter Kaufmann. New York: Simon and Schuster, 1996.

Bulka, Reuven P. *Jewish Marriage: A Halakhic Ethic.* New York: Ktav, 1986.

Butler, Judith. *Bodies that Matter: On the Discursive Limits of "Sex."* New York: Routledge, 1993.

Califia, Patrick. *Macho Sluts: A Little Sister's Classic.* Vancouver: Arsenal Pulp, 2009.

Carrette, Jeremy R. "Intense Exchange: Sadomasochism, Theology, and the Politics of Late Capitalism." *Theology and Sexuality* 11, no. 2 (2005): 11–30.

CDC—*see* Centers for Disease Control and Prevention

Centers for Disease Control and Prevention. "Burden of Foodborne Illness: Findings." Last modified November 5, 2018. https://www.cdc.gov /foodborneburden/2011-foodborne-estimates.html.

———. "Condoms and STDs: Fact Sheet for Public Health Personnel." Last modified September 14, 2021. https://www.cdc.gov/condomeffectiveness /latex.html.

———. "Genital Herpes—CDC Fact Sheet (Detailed)." Last modified July 22, 2021. https://www.cdc.gov/std/herpes/stdfact-herpes-detailed.htm.

———. "Pre-Exposure Prophylaxis (PrEP)." Last modified August 6, 2021. https://www.cdc.gov/hiv/risk/prep/index.html.

———. *Sexually Transmitted Disease Surveillance 2015.* Atlanta: US Department of Health and Human Services, 2016.

———. "2021 Sexually Transmitted Diseases Treatment Guidelines: Genital HSV Infections." Accessed June 2, 2022. https://www.cdc.gov/std/treatment -guidelines/herpes.htm.

Charania, Mahnaz R., Nicole Crepaz, Carolyn Guenther-Gray, Kirk Henny, Adrian Liau, Leigh A. Willis, and Cynthia M. Lyles. "Efficacy of Structural-Level Condom Distribution Interventions: A Meta-Analysis of U.S. and International Studies, 1998–2007." *AIDS and Behavior* 15 (2011): 1283–97. https:// doi.org/10.1007/s10461-010-9812-y.

Chow, Rey. "The Politics of Admittance." In *The Rey Chow Reader,* edited by Paul Bowman, 57–58. New York: Columbia University Press, 2010.

Chuang, Janie A. "Rescuing Trafficking from Ideological Capture: Prostitution Reform and Anti-Trafficking Law and Policy." *University of Pennsylvania Law Review* 158, no. 6 (2010): 1655–1728.

Clendinen, Dudley. "AIDS Spreads Pain and Fear among Ill and Healthy Alike." *New York Times*, June 17, 1983. http://www.nytimes.com/1983/06/17/us/aids -spreads-pain-and-fear-among-ill-and-healthy-alike.html.

Cohen, Shaye J. D. *From the Maccabees to the Mishnah*. 2nd ed. Louisville, KY: Westminster John Knox Press, 2006.

Colan, Jonathan D. "The Supreme Court's Talmudic Debate on the Meanings of Guilt, Innocence, and Finality." *Washington and Lee Law Review* 73, no. 1243 (June 2016). https://scholarlycommons.law.wlu.edu/wlulr/vol73 /iss3/8.

Cook, R. L., H. C. Wissenfeld, M. R. Ashton, M. A. Krohn, T. Zamborsky, and S. H. Scholle. "Barriers to Screening Sexually Active Adolescent Women for Chlamydia: A Survey of Primary Care Physicians." *Journal of Adolescent Health* 28 (2001): 204–10. https://doi.org/10.1016/s1054-139x(00)00152-x.

Cooke, Lucy J., Lucy C. Chambers, Elizabeth V. Añez, Helen A. Croker, David Boniface, Martin R. Yeomans, and Jane Wardle. "Eating for Pleasure or Profit: The Effect of Incentives on Children's Enjoyment of Vegetables." *Psychological Science* 22 (2011): 190–96. https://doi.org/10.1177/0956797610394662.

Cooper Owens, Deirdre. *Medical Bondage: Race, Gender, and the Origins of American Gynecology*. Athens: University of Georgia Press, 2017.

Corvid, Margaret. "Dear Jian Ghomeshi: Keep Your Abuse out of My Kink." Jezebel.com, October 28, 2014. https://jezebel.com/dear-jian-ghomeshi -keep-your-abuse-out-of-my-kink-1651373143.

Cruz, Ariane. *The Color of Kink: Black Women, BDSM, and Pornography*. New York: New York University Press, 2016.

Cutter, William, ed. *Midrash and Medicine: Healing Body and Soul in the Jewish Interpretive Tradition*. Woodstock, VT: Jewish Lights, 2011.

Deegan, Patricia E. "The Independent Living Movement and People with Psychiatric Disabilities: Taking Back Control over Our Own Lives." *Psychosocial Rehabilitation Journal* 15, no. 3 (January 1992): 3–19.

D'Emilio, John. *Sexual Politics, Sexual Communities: The Making of a Homosexual Minority in the United States, 1940–1970*. Chicago: University of Chicago Press, 1983.

DeJong, Gerben. "Independent Living: From Social Movement to Analytic Paradigm." *Archives of Physical Medicine and Rehabilitation* 60 (October 1979): 435–46.

Dewey, John. *Experience and Nature*. Chicago: Open Court, 1926.

Dohrman, Natalie B. "Reading as Rhetoric in Rabbinic Texts." In *Of Scribes and Sages: Early Jewish Interpretation and Transmission of Scripture*, vol. 2, edited by Craig A. Evans, 90–114. London: T&T Clark, 2004.

Dorff, Elliot. "A Jewish Perspective on Birth Control and Procreation." In *The Passionate Torah*, edited by Danya Ruttenberg, 152–68. New York: New York University Press, 2009.

——. "Judaism as a Religious Legal System." *Hastings Law Journal* 29, no. 1331 (1978). https://repository.uchastings.edu/hastings_law_journal/vol29/iss6/4.

——. *Love Your Neighbor and Yourself: A Jewish Approach to Modern Personal Ethics*. Philadelphia: Jewish Publication Society, 2003.

Douglas, Mary, and Aaron Wildavsky. *Risk and Culture: An Essay on the Selection of Technical and Environmental Dangers*. Berkeley: University of California Press, 1982.

Duggan, Lisa. "Down There: The Queer South and the Future of History Writing." *GLQ* 8, no. 3 (2002): 379–87.

Elliston, Deborah. "Anthropology's Queer Future: Feminist Lessons from Tahiti and Its Islands." In *Out in Theory: The Emergence of Lesbian and Gay Anthropology*, edited by Ellen Lewin and William Leap, 287–316. Urbana: University of Illinois Press, 2002.

Epstein-Levi, Rebecca J. "Is Judaism 'Sex Positive'? Understanding Trends in Recent Jewish Sexual Ethics." *G'vanim* 10 (2019): 14–34.

——. "A Polyvocal Body: Mutually Corrective Discourses in Feminist and Jewish Bodily Ethics." *Journal of Religious Ethics* 43, no. 2 (2015): 244–67.

——. "Textual Relationships: On Perspective, Interpretive Discipline, and Constructive Ethics." *Journal of Textual Reasoning* 10, no. 1 (2018). https://jtr.shanti.virginia.edu/vol-10-no-1-december-2018/textual-relationships-on-perspective-interpretive-discipline-and-constructive-ethics/.

Farber, Zev. "Extra-Legal Punishments in Medieval Jewish Courts." In *Mishpetei Shalom: A Jubilee Volume in Honor of Rabbi Saul (Shalom) Berman*, edited by Yamin Levy, 191–231. New York: Ktav, 2010.

Fildes, Alison, Cornelia H. M. van Jaarsveld, Jane Wardle, and Lucy Cooke. "A Randomized Controlled Trial of Parent-Administered Exposure to Increase Children's Vegetable Acceptance." *Journal of the Academy of Nutrition and Dietetics* 114, no. 6 (June 2014): 881–88. https://doi.org/10.1016/j.jand.2013.07.040.

Filler, Emily A. "Classical Rabbinic Literature and the Making of Jewish Ethics: A Formal Argument." Paper presented at the annual meeting of the Society for Jewish Ethics, Seattle, January 2014.

Flanagan, Bob, and Sheree Rose. *The Pain Journal*. Los Angeles: Semiotext(e), 2000.

Fletcher, Nichola. *Charlemagne's Tablecloth: A Piquant History of Feasting*. New York: St. Martin's, 2004.

Fonrobert, Charlotte. *Menstrual Purity: Rabbinic and Christian Reconstructions of Biblical Gender.* Stanford, CA: Stanford University Press, 2000.

Foucault, Michel. "Sexual Choice, Sexual Act." In *Foucault Live: Interviews, 1961–1984,* edited by Sylvère Lotringer, 322–34. Translated by Lysa Hochroth and John Johnston. New York: Semiotext(e), 1996.

Fredrickson, Barbara L., and Marcial F. Losada. "Positive Affect and the Complex Dynamics of Human Flourishing." *American Psychologist* 60, no. 7 (2005): 678–86. https://doi.org/10.1037/0003-066X.60.7.678.

Freedman, Benjamin. *Duty and Healing: Foundations of a Jewish Bioethic.* London: Routledge, 1999.

Frymer-Kensky, Tikva. "Pollution, Purification, and Purgation in Biblical Israel." In *The Word of the Lord Shall Go Forth: Essays in Honor of David Noel Freedman in Celebration of His Sixtieth Birthday,* edited by Carol Myers and M. O'Connor, 399–414. Winona Lake, IN: Eisenbrauns, 1983.

Furstenberg, Yair. *Ṭohorah u-ḳehilah ba-et ha-atiḳah: masorot ha-halakhah ben Yahadut Bayit Sheni la-Mishnah* [Purity and community in antiquity: Traditions of the law from Second Temple Judaism to the mishnah]. Jerusalem: Magnes, 2016.

Gaca, Kathy L. *The Making of Fornication: Eros, Ethics, and Political Reform in Greek Philosophy and Early Christianity.* Berkeley: University of California Press, 2017.

Gadamer, Hans-Georg. *Truth and Method.* 2nd rev. ed. Translated by Joel Weinsenheimer and Donald G. Marshall. London: Continuum, 2006.

Garnsey, Peter. "Why Penal Laws Become Harsher: The Roman Case." *Natural Law Forum* 143 (1968): 141–62.

Gilman, Sander. *The Jew's Body.* New York: Routledge, 1991.

Golub, Sarit A., Ja'Nina J. Walker, Buffie Longlmire-Avital, David S. Bimbi, and Jeffrey T. Parsons. "The Role of Religiosity, Social Support, and Stress-Related Growth in Protecting against HIV Risk among Transgender Women." *Journal of Health Psychology* 15, no. 8 (2010): 1135–44. https://doi.org/10.1177/1359105310364169.

Goodey, Jo. "Human Trafficking: Sketchy Data and Policy Responses." *Criminology and Criminal Justice* 8, no. 421 (2008). https://doi.org/10.1177/1748895808096471.

Gottlieb, Sami L., Nicola Low, Lori M. Newman, Gail Bolan, Mary Kamb, and Nathalie Brought. "Toward Global Prevention of Sexually Transmitted Infections STIs: The Need for STI Vaccines." *Vaccine* 32, no. 14 (March 2014): 1527–35. https://doi.org/10.1016/j.vaccine.2013.07.087.

Green, Arthur. "A Contemporary Approach to Jewish Sexuality." In *The Second Jewish Catalog: Sources and Resources,* edited by Michael Strassfeld and Sharon Strassfeld, 96–99. Philadelphia: Jewish Publication Society, 1976.

Greenberg, Steven. *Wrestling with God and Men: Homosexuality in the Jewish Tradition*. Madison: University of Wisconsin Press, 2004.

Groner, Rachel. "Sex as 'Spock': Autism, Sexuality, and Autobiographical Narrative." In *Sex and Disability*, edited by Robert McRuer and Anna Mollow, 263–84. Durham, NC: Duke University Press, 2012.

Halberstam, Chaya T. *Law and Truth in Biblical and Rabbinic Literature*. Bloomington: Indiana University Press, 2010.

Halbertal, Moshe. *Mahapekhot Parshaniyot Be-Hit'havutan: Arakhim Ke-Shiquilim Parshani'im Be-Midreshei Halakhah*. Jerusalem: Magnes, 1997.

Halwani, Raja, and Alan Soble, eds. *The Philosophy of Sex: Contemporary Readings*. 7th ed. Lanham, MD: Rowman and Littlefield, 2017.

Hamraie, Aimi. *Building Access: Universal Design and the Politics of Disability*. Minneapolis: University of Minnesota Press, 2017.

Hart, Mitchell B. *The Healthy Jew: The Symbiosis of Judaism and Modern Medicine*. Cambridge: Cambridge University Press, 2007.

Hayes, Christine E. *Gentile Impurities and Jewish Identities: Intermarriage and Conversion from the Bible to the Talmud*. Oxford: Oxford University Press, 2002.

Hayes, Christine, and Amos Israel-Vleeschhouwer, eds. *Jewish Law and Its Interaction with Other Legal Systems*. Liverpool: Deborah Charles Publications on behalf of the Jewish Law Association, 2014.

HIV Prevention Trial Network. "HPTN 052: A Randomized Trial to Evaluate the Effectiveness of Antiretroviral Therapy plus HIV Primary Care versus HIV Primary Care Alone to Prevent the Sexual Transmission of HIV-1 in Serodiscordant Couples." Accessed February 3, 2017. https://hptn.org/research/studies/33.

Hoffman, David Tzevi. *Das Buch Leviticus*. 2 vols. Berlin: M. Poppelauer, 1905–1906.

Hopkins, Patrick D. "Rethinking Sadomasochism: Feminism, Interpretation, and Simulation." *Hypatia* 9, no. 1 (1994): 116–41.

Imhoff, Sarah. "Jews, Sex Positivity, and Abuse." *The Revealer*, March 2, 2020. https://therevealer.org/jews-sex-positivity-and-abuse/.

Institute of Medicine. *The Hidden Epidemic: Confronting Sexually Transmitted Diseases*. Edited by Thomas R. Eng and William T. Butler. Washington, DC: National Academic Press, 2009. https://doi.org/10.17226/5284.

International Labour Organization. *Global Estimates of Modern Slavery: Forced Labour and Forced Marriage*. Geneva: International Labour Organization, 2017.

IOM—*see* Institute of Medicine

Jastrow, Marcus. *A Dictionary of the Targumim, the Talmud Babli and Yerushalmi, and the Midrashic Literature*. New York: G. Putnam's Sons, 1903.

Johanns, Karen. "Channels of Cum-munication, or Emotional Safety: A View from the Top." In *The Lesbian S/M Safety Manual*, edited by Patrick Califia, 5–12. Denver: Lace, 1988.

Joint United Nations Programme on HIV/AIDS. *The Gap Report 2014*. Geneva: UNAIDS, 2014.

———. *Global Report: UNAIDS Report on the Global AIDS Epidemic 2013*. Geneva: UNAIDS, 2013.

Jones, James H. *Bad Blood: The Tuskegee Syphilis Experiment*. 2nd ed. New York: Free Press, 1993.

Joseph, Miranda. *Against the Romance of Community*. Minneapolis: University of Minnesota Press, 2006.

Kafer, Alison. *Feminist, Queer, Crip*. Bloomington: Indiana University Press, 2013.

Kasperson, Roger E., Ortwin Renn, Paul Slovic, Halina S. Brown, Jacque Emel, Robert Goble, Jeanne X. Kasperson, and Samuel Ratick. "The Social Amplification of Risk: A Conceptual Framework." *Risk Analysis* 8, no. 2 (1988): 177–87.

Kepnes, Steven. *The Text as Thou: Martin Buber's Dialogical Hermeneutics and Narrative Theology*. Bloomington: Indiana University Press, 1992.

Kittay, Feder. *Love's Labor: Essays on Women, Equality, and Dependency*. New York: Routledge, 1999.

Klawans, Jonathan. *Impurity and Sin in Ancient Judaism*. Oxford: Oxford University Press, 2000.

Kukla, Rebecca. *Mass Hysteria: Medicine, Culture, and Mothers' Bodies*. Lanham, MD: Rowman and Littlefield, 2005.

Lacquer, Thomas. *Making Sex: Body and Gender from the Greeks to Freud*. Cambridge, MA: Harvard University Press, 1990.

Lamm, Maurice. *The Jewish Way in Love and Marriage*. Middle Village, NY: Jonathan David, 1991.

Leach Scully, Jackie. *Disability Bioethics: Moral Bodies, Moral Difference*. Lanham, MD: Rowman and Littlefield, 2008.

Levinas, Emanuel. *Totality and Infinity: An Essay on Exteriority*. Translated by Alphonso Lingis. Pittsburgh: Duquesne University Press, 1969.

Levine, Philippa. *Prostitution, Race, and Politics: Policing Venereal Disease in the British Empire*. London: Routledge, 2003.

Levine, Samuel J. "Capital Punishment in Jewish Law and Its Application to the American Legal System: A Conceptual Overview." *St. Mary's Law Journal* 29, no. 1037 (1998): 1037–38.

Linden, Robin Ruth, Darlene R. Pagano, Diana E. H. Russell, and Susan Leigh Star, eds. *Against Sadomasochism*. East Palo Alto, CA: Frog in the Well, 1982.

Longmire-Avital, Buffie. "'I Asked for the Papers': How Emerging Adult Black Women Request Sexual Health Information." *Journal of Black Sexuality and Relationships* 6, no. 1 (Summer 2019): 29–48. https://doi.org/10.1353/bsr.2019.0014.

Longmire-Avital, Buffie, and Virginia Oberle. "'Condoms Are the Standard, Right?': Exploratory Study of the Reasons for Using Condoms by Black American Emerging Adult Women." *Women and Health* 56, no. 2 (2016): 226–41. https://doi.org/10.1080/03630242.2015.1086469.

Looker, Katharine J., Amalia S. Magaret, Margaret T. May, Katherine M. E. Turner, Peter Vickerman, Sami L. Gottlieb, and Lori M. Newman. "Global and Regional Estimates of Prevalent and Incident Herpes Simplex Virus Type 1 Infections in 2012." *PLoS ONE* 10, no. 10 (October 2015). https://doi.org/10.1371/journal.pone.0140765.

Looker, Katharine J., Amalia S. Magaret, Katherine M. E. Turner, Peter Vickerman, Sami L. Gottlieb, and Lori M. Newman. "Global Estimates of Prevalent and Incident Herpes Simplex Virus Type 2 Infections in 2012." *PLoS ONE* 10, no. 1 (January 2015). https://doi.org/10.1371/journal.pone.0114989.

Lorberbaum, Yair. "Adam, Dam, Demut—Al Mitat Ha-Hereg Be-Sifrut Ha-Tannaim." *Bar-Ilan Law Studies* 15 (2000): 429–56.

———. "Tselem Elohim: Sifrut Hazal, Ha-Rambam, Ve-Ha-Ramban." PhD diss., Hebrew University, 1997.

Lorde, Audre. "Uses of the Erotic: The Erotic as Power." In *Sister Outsider: Essays and Speeches*, 53–59. Berkeley, CA: Crossings, 2007.

Luo, Rutao, Michael J. Piovoso, Javier Martinez-Picado, and Ryan Zurakowski. "Optimal Antiviral Switching to Minimize Resistance Risk in HIV Therapy." *PLOS One* 6, no. 11 (November 2011). https://doi.org/10.1371/journal.pone.0027047.

Lyerly, Anne Drapkin, Lisa M. Mitchell, Elizabeth Mitchell Armstrong, Lisa H. Harris, Rebecca Kukla, Miriam Kuppermann, and Margaret Olivia Little. "R I S K and the Pregnant Body." *Hastings Center Report* 39, no. 6 (November–December 2009): 34–42. https://www.jstor.org/stable/40407670.

Mabey, David. "Epidemiology of Sexually Transmitted Infections: Worldwide." *Medicine* 42, no. 6 (June 2014): 287–90. https://doi.org/10.1016/j.mpmed.2014.03.004.

MacIntyre, Alasdair. *After Virtue: A Study in Moral Theory*. 3rd ed. Notre Dame, IN: Notre Dame University Press, 2007.

MacKendrick, Karmen. *Counterpleasures*. Albany: State University of New York Press, 1999.

Magness, Jodi. *Stone and Dung, Oil and Spit: Jewish Daily Life in the Time of Jesus*. Grand Rapids, MI: Eerdmans, 2011.

Marcotte, Amanda. "The Jian Ghomeshi Accusations Are Not about BDSM. They Are about Consent." Slate.com, October 27, 2014. https://slate.com /human-interest/2014/10/jian-ghomeshi-accusations-against-the-q-host-are -not-about-bdsm-but-about-consent.html.

Martin, Biddy. "Extraordinary Homosexuals and the Fear of Being Ordinary." *Differences: A Journal of Feminist Cultural Studies* 6, no. 2–3 (1994): 100–126.

———. "Sexual Practice and Changing Lesbian Identities." In *Destabilizing Theory: Contemporary Feminist Debates*, edited by Michèle Barrett and Anne Phillips, 3–119. Stanford, CA: Stanford University Press, 1992.

McBryde Johnson, Harriet. "The Disability Gulag." *New York Times Magazine*, November 23, 2003.

McClintock, Anne. "Maid to Order: Commercial Feminism and Gender Power." *Social Text* 37 (1993): 87–116.

McElligott, Kara A. "Mortality from Sexually Transmitted Diseases in Reproductive-Aged Women: United States, 1999–2010." *American Journal of Public Health* 104, no. 8 (August 2014): e101–5. https://doi.org/10.2105 /AJPH.2014.302044.

McRuer, Robert. *Crip Theory: Cultural Signs of Queerness and Disability.* New York: New York University Press, 2006.

Mez, Jesse, Daniel H. Daneshvar, Patrick T. Kiernan, Bobak Abdolmohammadi, Victor E. Alvarez, Bertrand R. Huber, Michael L. Alosco, et al. "Clinicopathological Evaluation of Chronic Traumatic Encephalopathy in Players of American Football." *Journal of the American Medical Association* 318, no. 4 (July 2017): 360–70. https://doi.org/10.1001/jama.2017.8334.

Milgrom, J. "Sin-Offering or Purification-Offering?" *Vetus Testamentum* 21 (1971): 237–39.

Milgrom, Jacob. *Leviticus 1–16. A New Translation with Introduction and Commentary.* Vol. 3 of *The Anchor Bible.* New York: Doubleday, 1992.

Miller, Stuart. *At the Intersection of Texts and Material Finds: Stepped Pools, Stone Vessels, and Ritual Purity among the Jews of Roman Galilee.* Gottingen, Ger.: Vandenhoeck & Ruprecht, 2015.

Millstein, Susan G., Vivien Igra, and Janet Gans. "Delivery of STD/HIV Preventive Services to Adolescents by Primary Care Physicians." *Journal of Adolescent Health* 19 (1996): 249–57. https://doi.org/10.1016/S1054-139X9600092-4.

Mingus, Mia. "Access Intimacy: The Missing Link." *Leaving Evidence,* May 5, 2011. https://leavingevidence.wordpress.com/2011/05/05/access -intimacy-the-missing-link/.

———. "Forced Intimacy: An Ableist Norm." *Leaving Evidence,* August 6, 2017. https://leavingevidence.wordpress.com/2017/08/06/forced-intimacy -an-ableist-norm/.

Minkoff, Howard, and Mary Faith Marshall. "Fetal Risks, Relative Risks, and Relatives' Risks." *American Journal of Bioethics* 16, no. 2 (February 2016): 3–11. https://doi.org/10.1080/15265161.2015.1120791.

Mullin, Amy. *Reconceiving Pregnancy and Childcare: Ethics, Experience, and Reproductive Labor.* Cambridge: Cambridge University Press, 2005.

Muñoz, José Esteban. *Cruising Utopia: The Then and There of Queer Futurity.* New York: New York University Press, 2009.

———. *Disidentifications: Queers of Color and the Performance of Politics.* Minneapolis: University of Minnesota, 1999.

Musser, Amber Jamilla. *Sensational Flesh: Race, Power, and Masochism.* New York: New York University Press, 2014.

Nash, Jennifer. *The Black Body in Ecstasy: Reading Race, Reading Pornography.* Durham, NC: Duke University Press, 2014.

National Library of Medicine. "Visual Culture and Public Health Posters: Venereal Disease." History of Medicine. Last modified September 8, 2011. https://www.nlm.nih.gov/exhibition/visualculture/venereal.html.

Neis, R. R. *The Sense of Sight in Rabbinic Culture: Jewish Ways of Seeing in Late Antiquity.* Cambridge: Cambridge University Press, 2013.

Nelson, James. *Embodiment: An Approach to Sexuality and Christian Theology.* Minneapolis: Augsburg, 1978.

Newmahr, Staci. *Playing on the Edge: Sadomasochism, Risk, and Intimacy.* Bloomington: Indiana University Press, 2011.

Newman, Louis E. "Woodchoppers and Respirators: The Problem of Interpretation in Contemporary Jewish Ethics." In *Contemporary Jewish Ethics and Morality: A Reader,* edited by Elliot N. Dorff and Louis E. Newman, 140–60. Oxford: Oxford University Press, 1995.

Novak, David. *Jewish Justice: The Contested Limits of Nature, Law, and Covenant.* Waco, TX: Baylor University Press, 2017.

———. *Jewish Social Ethics.* Oxford: Oxford University Press, 1992.

Nussbaum, Martha. *Upheavals of Thought: The Intelligence of Emotions.* Cambridge: Cambridge University Press, 2003.

———. "'Whether from Reason or Prejudice': Taking Money for Bodily Services." In *Sex and Social Justice,* 276–98. Oxford: Oxford University Press, 1999.

Oriel, J. David. *The Scars of Venus: A History of Venereology.* London: Springer-Verlag, 1994.

Paix, B. R. "Rider Injury Rates and Emergency Medical Services at Equestrian Events." *British Journal of Sports Medicine* 33 (February 1999): 46–48. https://doi.org/10.1136/bjsm.33.1.46.

Parascandola, John. *Sex, Sin, and Science: A History of Syphilis in America.* Westport, CT: Praeger, 2008.

Pava, Moses. *Jewish Ethics in a Post-Madoff World: A Case for Optimism.* New York: Palgrave Macmillan, 2011.

Perry, David M., and Lawrence Carter-Long. *The Ruderman White Paper on Media Coverage of Law Enforcement Use of Force and Disability.* Boston: Ruderman Family Foundation, 2016. https://rudermanfoundation.org/white_papers/media-coverage-of-law-enforcement-use-of-force-and-disability/.

Perske, Robert. "The Dignity of Risk and the Mentally Retarded." *Mental Retardation* 10, no. 1 (1972): 25–27.

Pierce, Jenelle Marie. "What Is Safer Sex—a Comprehensive Approach." The STI Project. Last modified June 4, 2020. https://thestiproject.com/what-is-safer-sex/.

Planned Parenthood. "Safer Sex ('Safe Sex') | Reduce Your Risk of Getting STDs." Accessed March 17, 2017. https://www.plannedparenthood.org/learn/stds-hiv-safer-sex/safer-sex.

Plaskow, Judith, and Donna Berman, ed. *The Coming of Lilith: Essays on Feminism, Judaism, and Sexual Ethics, 1972–2003.* Boston: Beacon, 2005.

Presner, Todd Samuel. *Muscular Judaism: The Jewish Body and the Politics of Regeneration.* New York: Routledge, 2007.

Quetel, Claude. *A History of Syphilis.* Translated by Judith Braddock and Brian Pike. Baltimore: Johns Hopkins University Press, 1990.

Raucher, Michal S. "Ethnography and Jewish Ethics: Lessons from a Case Study in Reproductive Ethics." *Journal of Religious Ethics* 44, no. 4 (2016): 636–58.

Reid-Pharr, Robert. *Black Gay Man: Essays.* New York: New York University Press, 2001.

Remington, Anna, Elizabeth Añez, Helen Croker, Jane Wardle, and Lucy Cooke. "Increasing Food Acceptance in the Home Setting: A Randomized Controlled Trial of Parent-Administered Taste Exposure with Incentives." *American Journal of Clinical Nutrition* 95 (2011): 72–77.

Ribner, David S., and Jennie Rosenfeld. *Et Le'ehov: The Newlywed's Guide to Sexual Intimacy.* Jerusalem: Gefen, 2011.

Rich, Adrienne. "Compulsory Heterosexuality and Lesbian Existence." *Signs: Journal of Women in Culture and Society* 5, no. 4 (1980): 631–60.

Roberts, Dorothy E. *Killing the Black Body: Race, Reproduction, and the Meaning of Liberty.* 2nd ed. New York: Vintage Books, 2016.

Rosenfeld, Jennie. "Talmudic Re-readings: Toward a Modern Orthodox Sexual Ethic." PhD diss., City University of New York, 2008.

Rosen-Zvi, Ishay. *The Mishnaic Sotah Ritual: Temple, Gender, and Midrash.* Leiden, Neth.: Brill, 2012.

Rouselle, Aline. *Porneia: On the Body and Desire in Antiquity.* Translated by Felicia Pheasant. Eugene, OR: Wipf & Stock, 1988.

Rubenstein, Jeffrey L. *The Culture of the Babylonian Talmud*. Baltimore: Johns Hopkins University Press, 2003.

Rubin, Gayle. "Old Guard, New Guard." *Cuir* 4, no. 2 (Summer 1998). http://black-rose.com/cuiru/archive/4-2/oldguard.html.

———. "Thinking Sex: Notes for a Radical Theory of the Politics of Sexuality." In *Pleasure and Danger: Exploring Female Sexuality*, edited by Carole S. Vance, 267–319. Boston: Routledge and Kegan Paul, 1984.

Russell, Bertrand. *Marriage and Morals*. New York: Horace Liveright, 1929.

Ruttenberg, Danya. "Jewish Sexual Ethics." In *The Oxford Handbook of Jewish Ethics and Morality*, edited by Elliot N. Dorff and Jonathan K. Crane, 383–400. Oxford: Oxford University Press, 2013.

———, ed. *The Passionate Torah: Sex and Judaism*. New York: New York University Press, 2009.

Ryan, Christopher, and Cacilda Jetha. *Sex at Dawn: How We Mate, Why We Stray, and What It Means for Modern Relationships*. New York: HarperCollins, 2010.

Sandahl, Carrie. "Queering the Crip or Cripping the Queer? Intersections of Queer and Crip Identities in Solo Autobiographical Performance." *GLQ: A Journal of Lesbian and Gay Studies* 9, no. 1–2 (2003): 25–56.

Sandel, Michael. *Liberalism and the Limits of Justice*. 2nd ed. Cambridge: Cambridge University Press, 1998.

Satlow, Michael. *Tasting the Dish: Rabbinic Rhetorics of Sexuality*. Providence, RI: Brown Judaic Studies, 1995.

Savage, Dan. "Magnum Episode #365." *Savage Lovecast*, October 22, 2013. Podcast, 44:47. http://www.savagelovecast.com/episodes/365#.WJSiI7badE4.

Schader, Susan M., and Mark A. Wainberg. "Insights into HIV-1 Pathogenesis through Drug Discovery: 30 Years of Basic Research and Concerns for the Future." *HIV and AIDS Review* 10, no. 4 (December 2011): 91–98.

Schofer, Jonathan Wyn. *Confronting Vulnerability: The Body and the Divine in Rabbinic Ethics*. Chicago: University of Chicago Press, 2010.

———. *The Making of a Sage: A Study in Rabbinic Ethics*. Madison: University of Wisconsin Press, 2005.

Scott, Catherine. *Thinking Kink: The Collision of BDSM, Feminism, and Popular Culture*. Jefferson, NC: McFarland, 2015.

Scott, James C. *Domination and the Arts of Resistance: Hidden Transcripts*. New Haven, CT: Yale University Press, 1990.

Sedgewick, Eve Kosofsky. *Epistemology of the Closet*. Berkeley: University of California Press, 1990.

Seltzer, Sarah. "A Feminist BDSM Expert Weighs in on Jian Ghomeshi." Flavorwire.com, October 30, 2014. http://flavorwire.com/485559/a-feminist-bdsm-expert-weighs-in-on-jian-ghomeshi.

Shanks Alexander, Elizabeth. "Ancient Jewish Gender." In *Early Judaism: New Insights and Scholarship*, edited by Frederick E. Greenspahn, 174–98. New York: New York University Press, 2018.

———. *Gender and Timebound Commandments in Judaism*. Cambridge: Cambridge University Press, 2013.

Shemesh, Aharon. *Onashim ve-ḥata'im: min ha-Miḳra le-sifrut ḥaza"l* [Punishments and sins from scripture to the rabbis]. Jerusalem: Magnes, 2003.

Silberman, Steve. *Neurotribes: The Legacy of Autism and the Future of Neurodiversity*. New York: Avery, 2015.

Singer, Judy. "'Why Can't You Be Normal for Once in Your Life?' From a 'Problem with No Name' to the Emergence of a New Category of Difference." In *Disability Discourse*, edited by Marian Corker and Sally French, 59–67. Buckingham, UK: Open University Press, 1999.

Sisson, Kathy. "The Cultural Formation of S/M: History and Analysis." In *Safe, Sane, and Consensual: Contemporary Perspectives on Sadomasochism*, edited by Darren Langdridge and Meg-John Barker, 16–40. New York: Palgrave Macmillan, 2007.

Smith, Leah H., J. S. Kaufman, Erin C. Strumpf, and Linda E. Lévesque. "Effects of Human Papillomavirus HPV Vaccination on Clinical Indicators of Sexual Behavior among Adolescent Girls: The Ontario Grade 8 HPV Vaccine Cohort Study." *Canadian Medical Association Journal* 187, no. 2 (February 2015): e74–e81. https://doi.org/10.1503/cmaj.140900.

Spencer, Ruth. "What I Know about Jian Ghomeshi." TheCut.com, September 15, 2018. https://www.thecut.com/2018/09/jian-ghomeshi-new-york-review-of-books-essay.html.

stein, david. "Safe, Sane, Consensual: The Making of a Shibboleth." 2002. Accessed March 13, 2019. http://www.boybear.us/ssc.pdf (site discontinued).

Steinmetz, Devora. "Crimes and Punishments, Part I: Mitot Beit Din as a Reflection of Rabbinic Jurisprudence." *Journal of Jewish Studies* 55 (2004): 81–101.

———. "Crimes and Punishments, Part II: Noachide Law, Brother-Sister Intercourse, and the Case of Murder." *Journal of Jewish Studies* 55 (2004): 278–305.

St. Lawrence, Janet S., Daniel E. Montaño, Danuta Kasprzyk, William R. Phillips, Keira Armstrong, and Jami S. Leichliter. "STI Screening, Testing, Case Reporting, and Clinical and Partner Notification Practices: A National Survey of US Physicians." *American Journal of Public Health* 92, no. 11 (2002): 1784–88. https://doi.org/10.2105/ajph.92.11.1784.

Stoeffel, Kat. "Jian Ghomeshi Isn't the First Alleged Abuser to Cite the Right to BDSM Sexuality." TheCut.com, October 28, 2014. https://www.thecut.com/2014/10/jian-ghomeshi-and-the-right-to-bdsm-sexuality.html.

Stone, Suzanne Last. "In Pursuit of the Counter-Text: The Turn to the Jewish Legal Model in Contemporary American Legal Theory." *Harvard Law Review* 106, no. 4 (1993): 813–94.

Switch, Gary. "Origin of RACK: RACK vs. SSC." *Prometheus* 37 (2011). https://www.the-iron-gate.com/essays/138.

Taormino, Tristan. "'S is for . . .': The Terms, Principles, and Pleasures of Kink." In *The Ultimate Guide to Kink: BDSM, Role Play, and the Erotic Edge*, edited by Tristan Taormino, 3–32. Berkeley, CA: Cleis, 2012.

Teutsch, David. *A Guide to Jewish Practice*. Vol. 1, *Everyday Living*. Wyncote, PA: RRC Press, 2011.

UNAIDS. "Fact Sheet." Accessed June 28, 2015. http://www.unaids.org/en/resources/campaigns/globalreport2013/factsheet.

US Fire Administration. "U.S. Fire Statistics." Accessed April 15, 2019. https://www.usfa.fema.gov/data/statistics/.

Vonlehrer, R. A., and J. R. Heller Jr. "The New Attack on Venereal Disease." *Science Illustrated* (January 1949): 29–30, 99. https://web.archive.org/web/20210120013343/http://blog.modernmechanix.com/the-new-attack-on-venereal-disease/.

Wald, Anna, and Lawrence Corey. "Persistence in the Population: Epidemiology, Transmission." In *Human Herpesviruses: Biology, Therapy, and Immunoprophylaxis*, edited by Ann Arvin, Gabriella Campadelli-Fiume, Edward Mocarski, Patrick S. Moore, Bernard Roizman, Richard Whitley, and Koichi Yamanishi. Cambridge: Cambridge University Press, 2007. https://www.ncbi.nlm.nih.gov/books/NBK47447/.

Walker, Ja'Nina J., Buffie Longmire-Avital, and Sarit Golub. "Racial and Sexual Identities as Potential Buffers to Risky Sexual Behavior for Black Gay and Bisexual Emerging Adult Men." *Health Psychology* 34, no. 8 (2015): 841–46. https://doi.org/10.1037/hea0000187.

Washington, Harriet A. *Medical Apartheid: The Dark History of Medical Experimentation on African Americans from Colonial Times to the Present*. New York: Doubleday, 2006.

Wasserman, Mira. *Jews, Gentiles, and Other Animals: The Talmud after the Humanities*. Philadelphia: University of Pennsylvania Press, 2017.

Watts Belser, Julia. "Brides and Blemishes: Queering Women's Disability in Rabbinic Marriage Law." *Journal of the American Academy of Religion* 84, no. 2 (2016): 401–29. https://doi.org/10.1093/jaarel/lfv070.

Weiss, Margot. *Techniques of Pleasure: BDSM and the Circuits of Sexuality*. Durham, NC: Duke University Press, 2011.

Welch, Sharon D. *A Feminist Ethic of Risk*. Minneapolis: Fortress, 1990.

Wendell, Susan. "Unhealthy Disabled: Treating Chronic Illness as Disability."
    Hypatia 16, no. 4 (2001): 31.

WHO—*see* World Health Organization

Wiedemann, Thomas E. J. *Emperors and Gladiators.* New York: Routledge, 1992.

Williams, Mollenna. "BDSM and Playing with Race." In *Best Sex Writing 2010,*
    edited by Rachel Kramer Bussel, 60–79. San Francisco: Cleis, 2010.

Winkler, Ethan A., John K. Yue, John F. Burke, Andrew K. Chan, Sanjay S.
    Dhall, Mitchel S. Berger, Geoffrey T. Manley, and Phiroz E. Tarapore. "Adult
    Sports-Related Traumatic Brain Injury in United States Trauma Centers."
    Neurosurgical Focus 40, no. 4 (April 2016): e4. https://doi.org/10.3171/2016.1.F
    OCUS15613.

Wiseman, Jay. *SM 101: A Realistic Introduction.* 2nd ed. San Francisco: Greenery,
    1998.

Wolpert, Julian. "The Dignity of Risk." *Transactions of the Institute of British
    Geographers* 5, no. 4 (1980): s391–401.

World Health Organization. "Global Health Observatory Data." Accessed June
    8, 2015. http://www.who.int/gho/hiv/en/.

———. *Global Incidence and Prevalence of Selected Curable Sexually Transmitted
    Infections—2008.* Geneva: World Health Organization, 2012.

———. "Herpes Simplex Virus." May 1, 2020. https://www.who.int/news-room
    /fact-sheets/detail/herpes-simplex-virus.

Wyn Schofer, Jonathan. *The Making of a Sage: A Study in Rabbinic Ethics.* Madi-
    son: University of Wisconsin Press, 2005.

Yadin, Azzan. *Scripture as Logos: Rabbi Ishmael and the Origins of Midrash.* Phila-
    delphia: University of Pennsylvania Press, 2004.

Zisk, Alyssa. "I Hid." In *Loud Hands: Autistic People, Speaking,* edited by Julia
    Bascom, 189–91. Washington, DC: Autistic Press, 2012.

Zoloth, Laurie. *Healthcare and the Ethics of Encounter: A Jewish Discussion of
    Social Justice.* Chapel Hill: University of North Carolina Press, 1999.

INDEX

Rebecca J. Epstein-Levi is Assistant Professor of Jewish Studies and Gender and Sexuality Studies at Vanderbilt University. An expert on sexual ethics, she uses unconventional readings of classical rabbinic text to study the ethics of sex and sexuality, disability, and neurodiversity. In her copious free time, she enjoys cooking unnecessarily complicated meals and sharpening her overly large collection of kitchen knives. She lives with her wife, Sarah; her cats, Faintly Macabre and Chroma the Great; and a rapidly expanding flock of wire dinosaurs and other beasties. You can follow her on Twitter @RJELevi.